Let's talk about your brain.

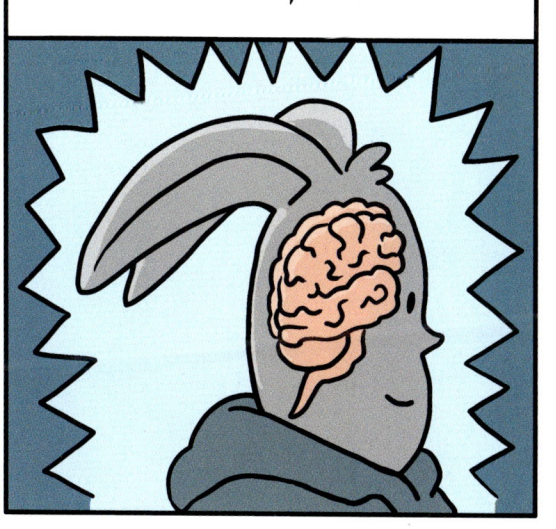

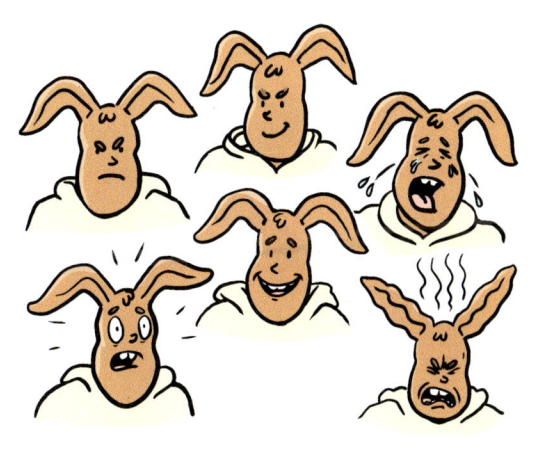

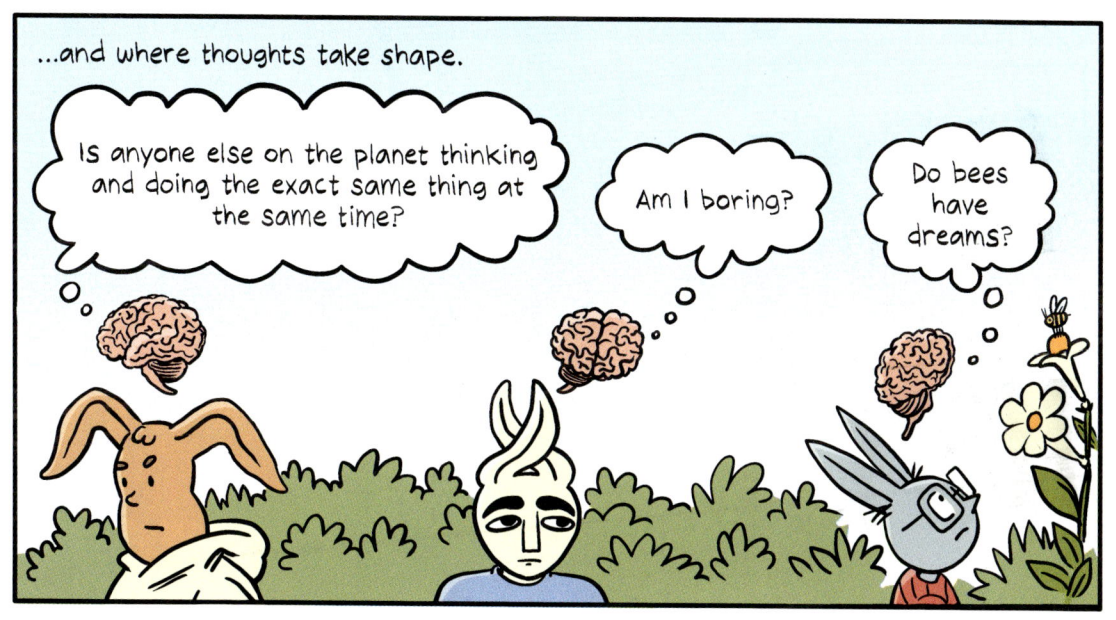

It's a place where emotions begin...

...and where thoughts take shape.

Is anyone else on the planet thinking and doing the exact same thing at the same time?

Am I boring?

Do bees have dreams?

Sometimes our brains are going to create upsetting emotions and negative thoughts.

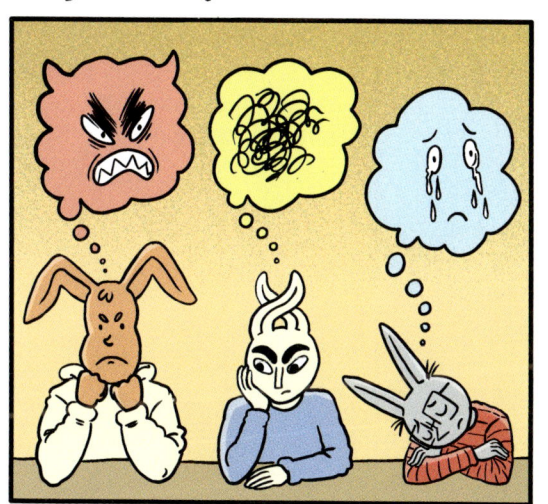

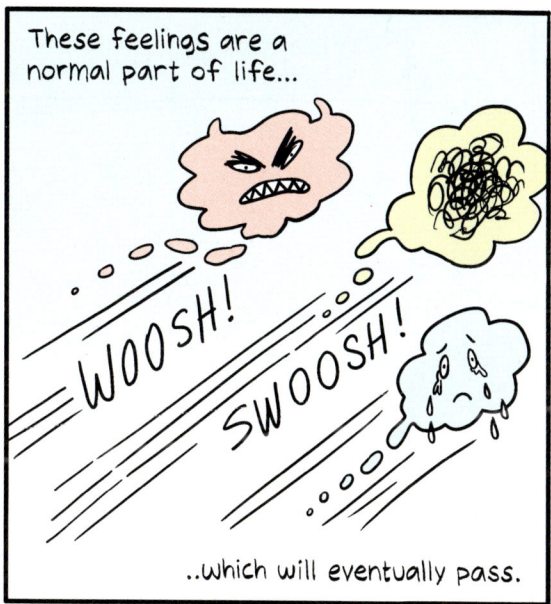

These feelings are a normal part of life...

WOOSH! SWOOSH!

..which will eventually pass.

WHAT IS STRESS?

Is stress a feeling of being pulled in too many directions?

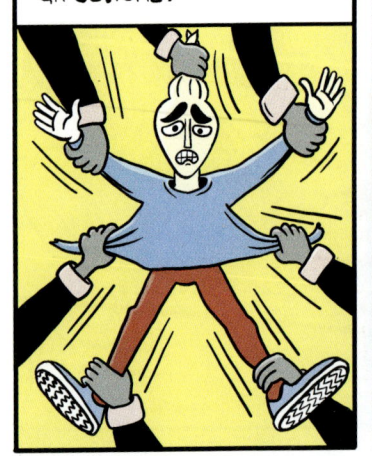

Is stress the pressure of daily life weighing you down?

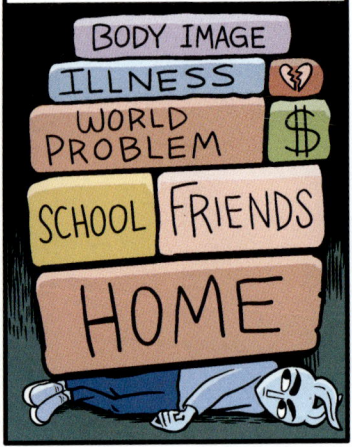

BODY IMAGE
ILLNESS
WORLD PROBLEM
$
SCHOOL FRIENDS
HOME

Or is stress a presence lurking in the background as you go about your day?

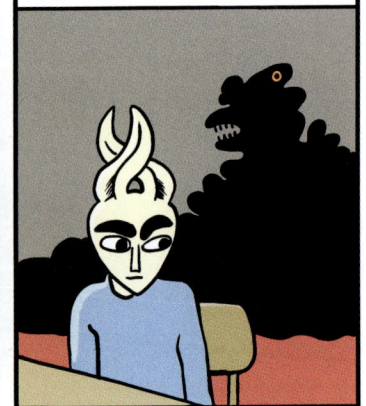

Stress is mental or emotional strain. This is something everyone experiences.

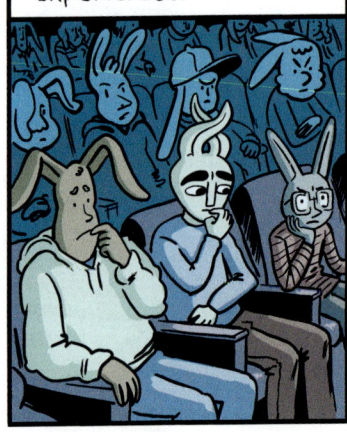

It can cause physical changes in the body...

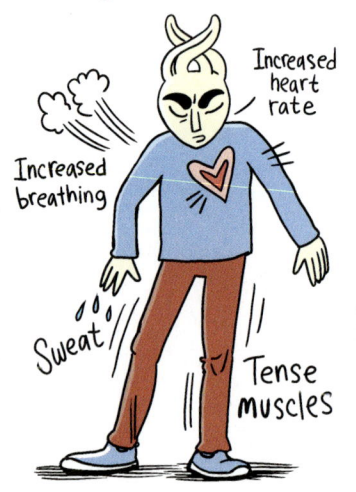

Increased breathing
Increased heart rate
Sweat
Tense muscles

...and in short bursts can actually be a good thing.

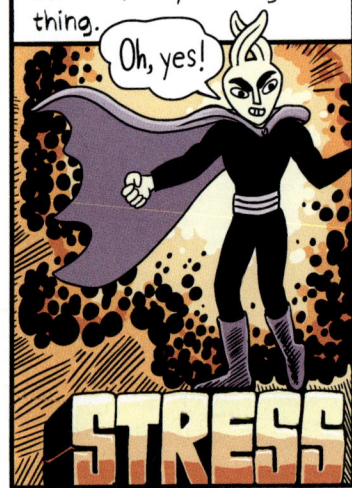

Oh, yes!

STRESS

The stress response has evolved to keep us safe.

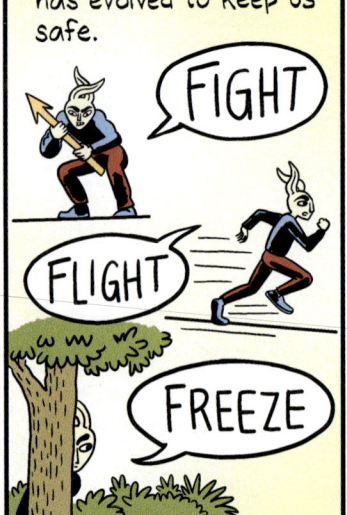

FIGHT
FLIGHT
FREEZE

Research shows that thinking skills improve as stress increases.

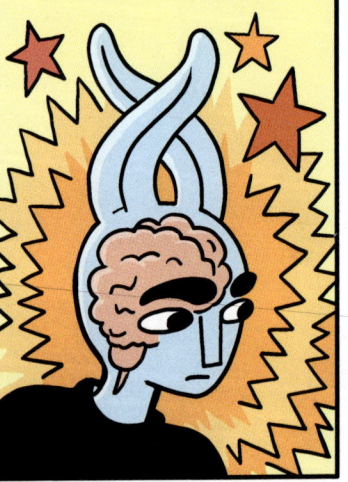

It can help us prepare for a performance, exam, or athletic competition. Usually, after a stressful event, the body returns to its normal state.

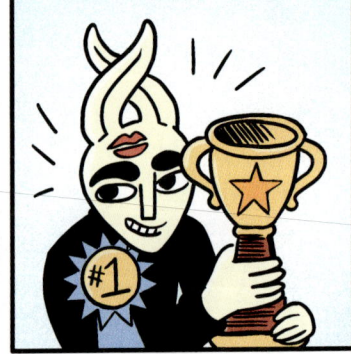

#1

TALKING ABOUT MENTAL HEALTH CAN BE WEIRD

And what does it even mean to be mentally healthy?

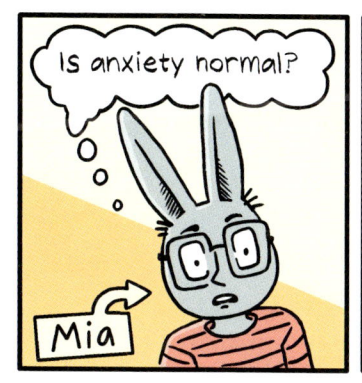

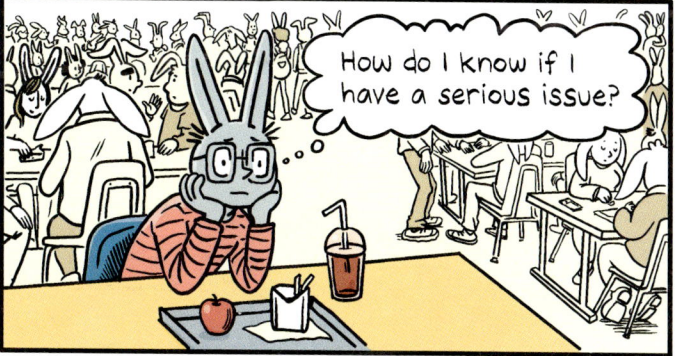

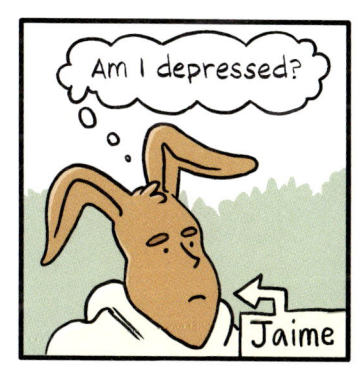

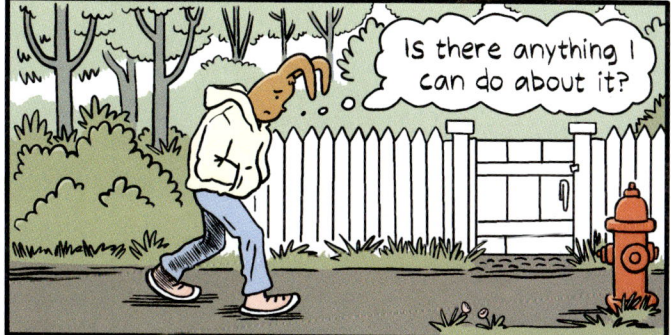

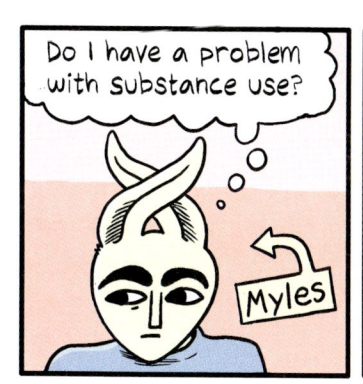

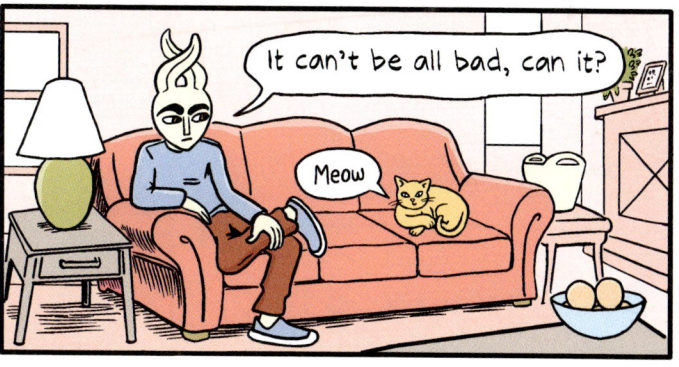

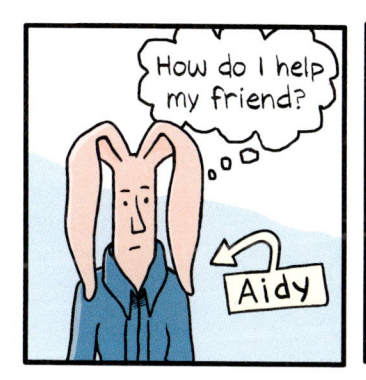

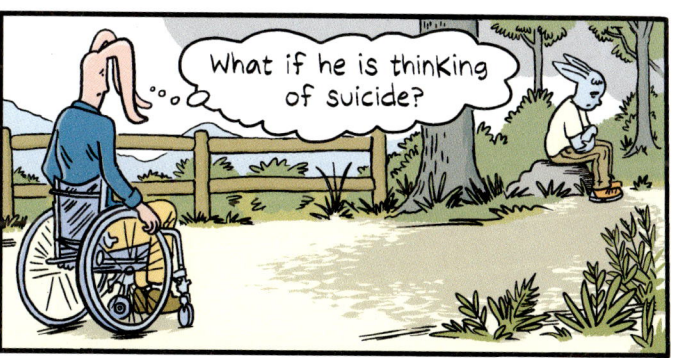

Mia: Is anxiety normal? How do I know if I have a serious issue?

Jaime: Am I depressed? Is there anything I can do about it?

Myles: Do I have a problem with substance use? It can't be all bad, can it?

Meow

Aidy: How do I help my friend? What if he is thinking of suicide?

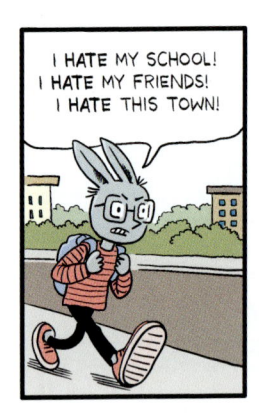

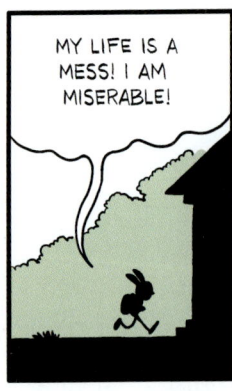

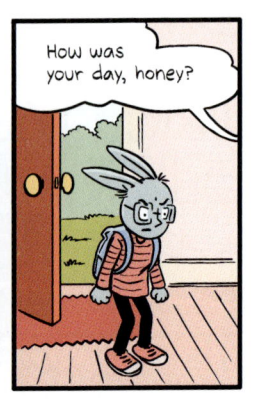

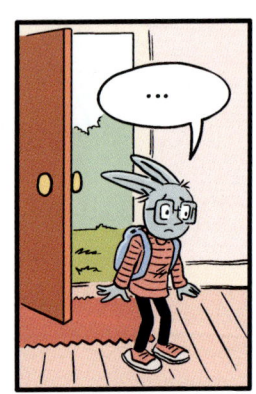

EMOTIONS CAN BE HARD TO TALK ABOUT, PARTLY BECAUSE OF STIGMA.

A stigma is a negative label that sets a person apart from others and leads to discrimination.

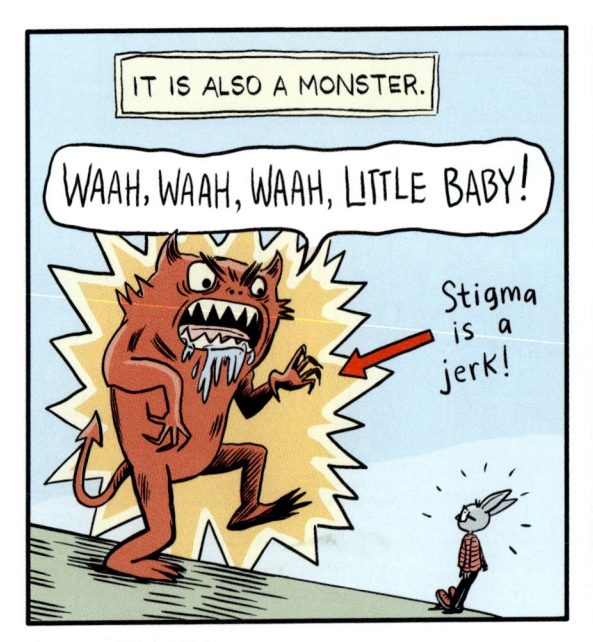

IT IS ALSO A MONSTER.

"WAAH, WAAH, WAAH, LITTLE BABY!"

Stigma is a jerk!

Stigma can make it harder for people to share their emotions.

"YOU CAN'T ESCAPE ME! I'M IN SOCIETY! I'M EVERYWHERE!"

Gulp!

When we buy into these stigmas and stereotypes, we can develop shame and low self-esteem.

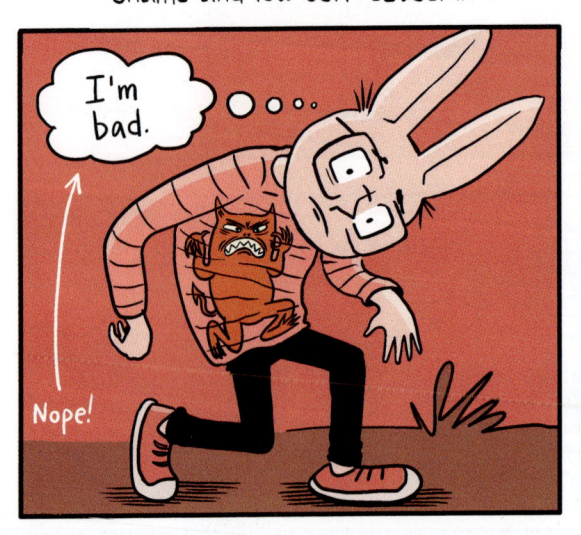

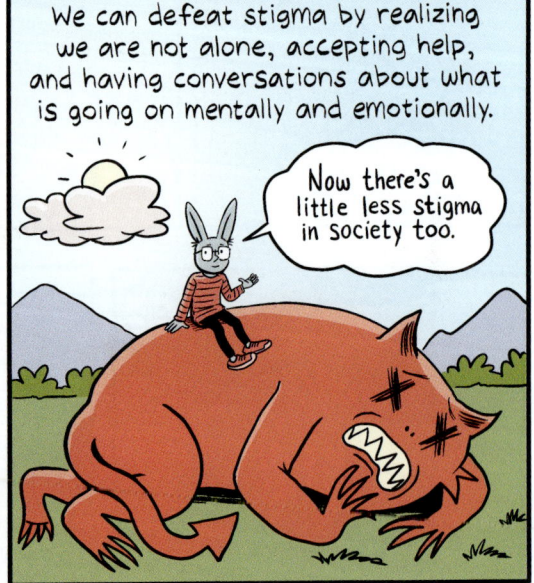

"I'm bad."

Nope!

We can defeat stigma by realizing we are not alone, accepting help, and having conversations about what is going on mentally and emotionally.

"Now there's a little less stigma in society too."

WHAT TO DO WITH STRESS

It is not good to be stressed all the time.

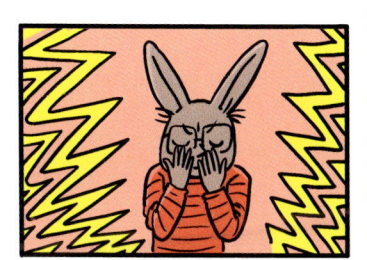

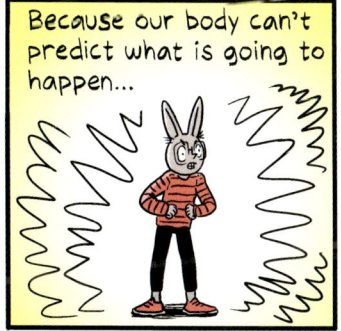

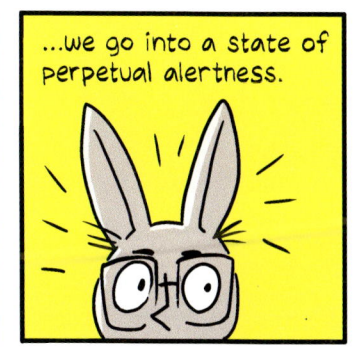

Because our body can't predict what is going to happen...

...we go into a state of perpetual alertness.

If we aren't able to calm our body and brain, then this can cause problems.

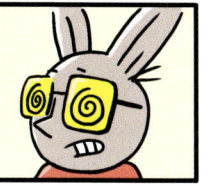

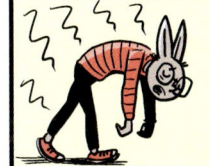

Stress can make us physically and mentally sick!

There are many healthy ways to manage stress.

- Be in nature
- Breathe
- Make art
- Talk to someone you trust
- Exercise
- Make music
- Yoga
- Clean and organize
- Spend time with pets
- Make food
- Listen to music
- Dance
- Write about it
- Laugh
- Read

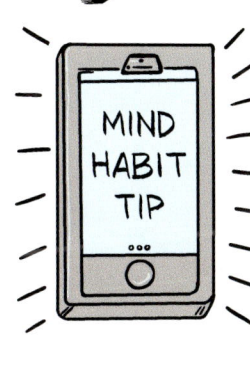

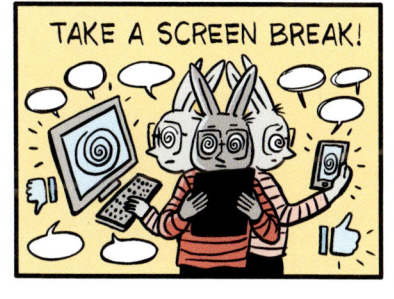

MIND HABIT TIP

TAKE A SCREEN BREAK!

Using social media more than three hours a day can increase feelings of depression, anxiety, poor body image, loneliness, and stress.

REST.

STRESS AND SLEEP!

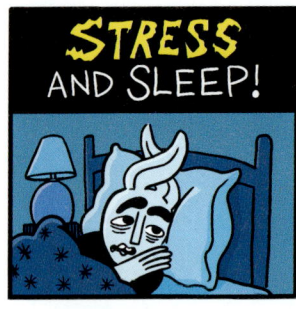

Why does lack of sleep make life harder?

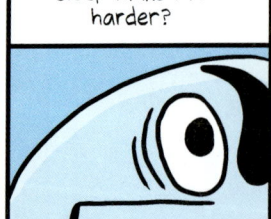

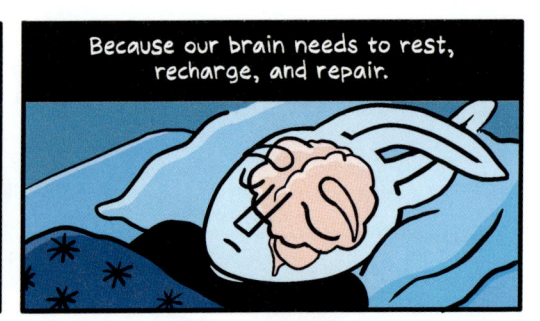

Because our brain needs to rest, recharge, and repair.

Lack of sleep affects memory and concentration and can lead to...

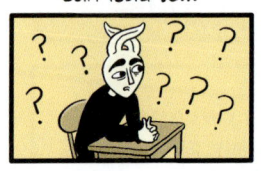

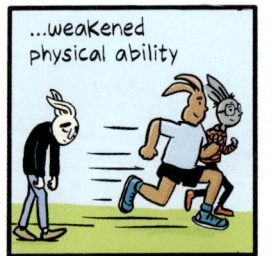

...weakened physical ability

...skin issues like acne

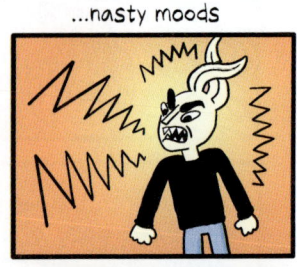

...nasty moods

...bad eating habits

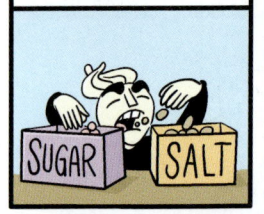

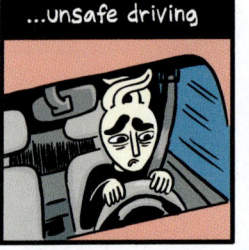

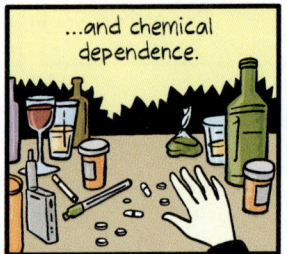

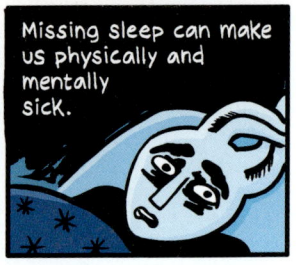

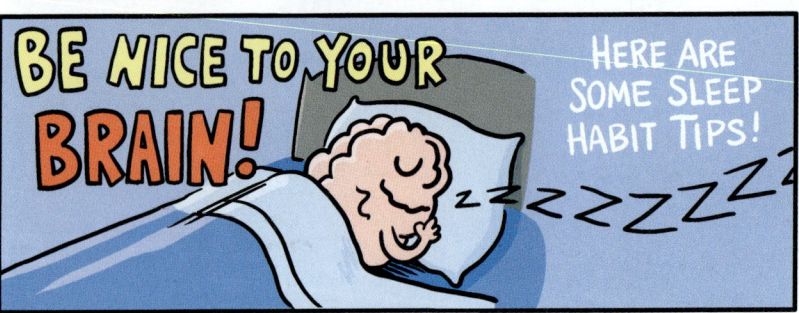

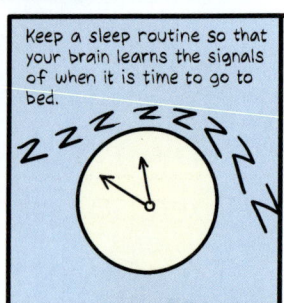

...unsafe driving

...and chemical dependence.

Missing sleep can make us physically and mentally sick.

BE NICE TO YOUR BRAIN!

HERE ARE SOME SLEEP HABIT TIPS!

Keep a sleep routine so that your brain learns the signals of when it is time to go to bed.

At bedtime, try taking a bath or shower (this will leave you extra time in the morning).

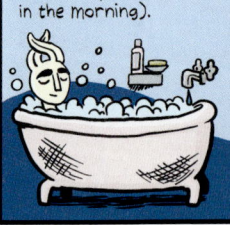

Avoid the T.V., computer, and your phone before you go to bed. (Blue light from screens disrupts sleep) Try reading a book instead.

Stay away from coffee, tea, soda/pop, and chocolate late in the day. (Nicotine and alcohol also interfere with sleep.)

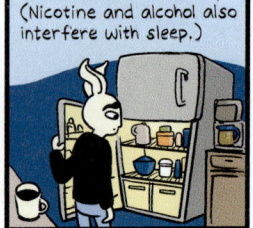

If you find yourself worrying or unable to stop your thoughts enough to relax, grab a notebook or a journal to create a to-do list or just to get your thoughts down on paper and out of your mind.

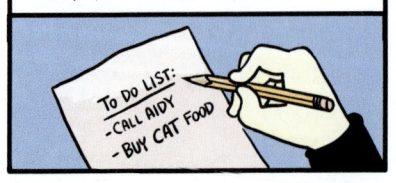

Make your sleep space a safe haven. Keep it cool, quiet, and dark.

Establish a bedtime and waketime and stick to it.

Try to stick to your schedule (or as close as you can) on weekends too.

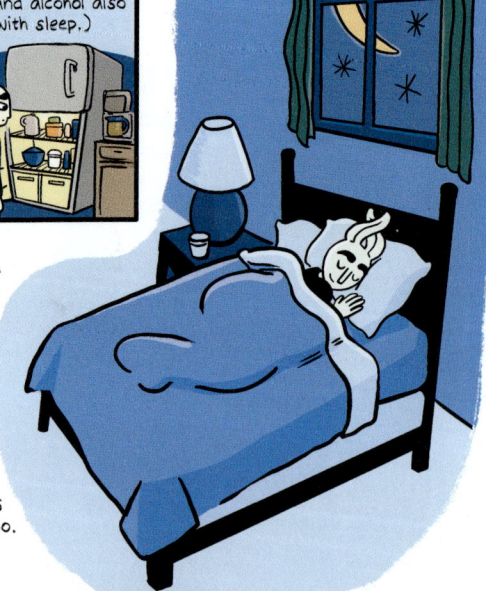

To Do List:
- CALL AIDY
- BUY CAT FOOD

8

MINDFULNESS IS A STRESS-FIGHTING SUPER POWER

Focusing on the present, the here and now, without judgment can help ground you.

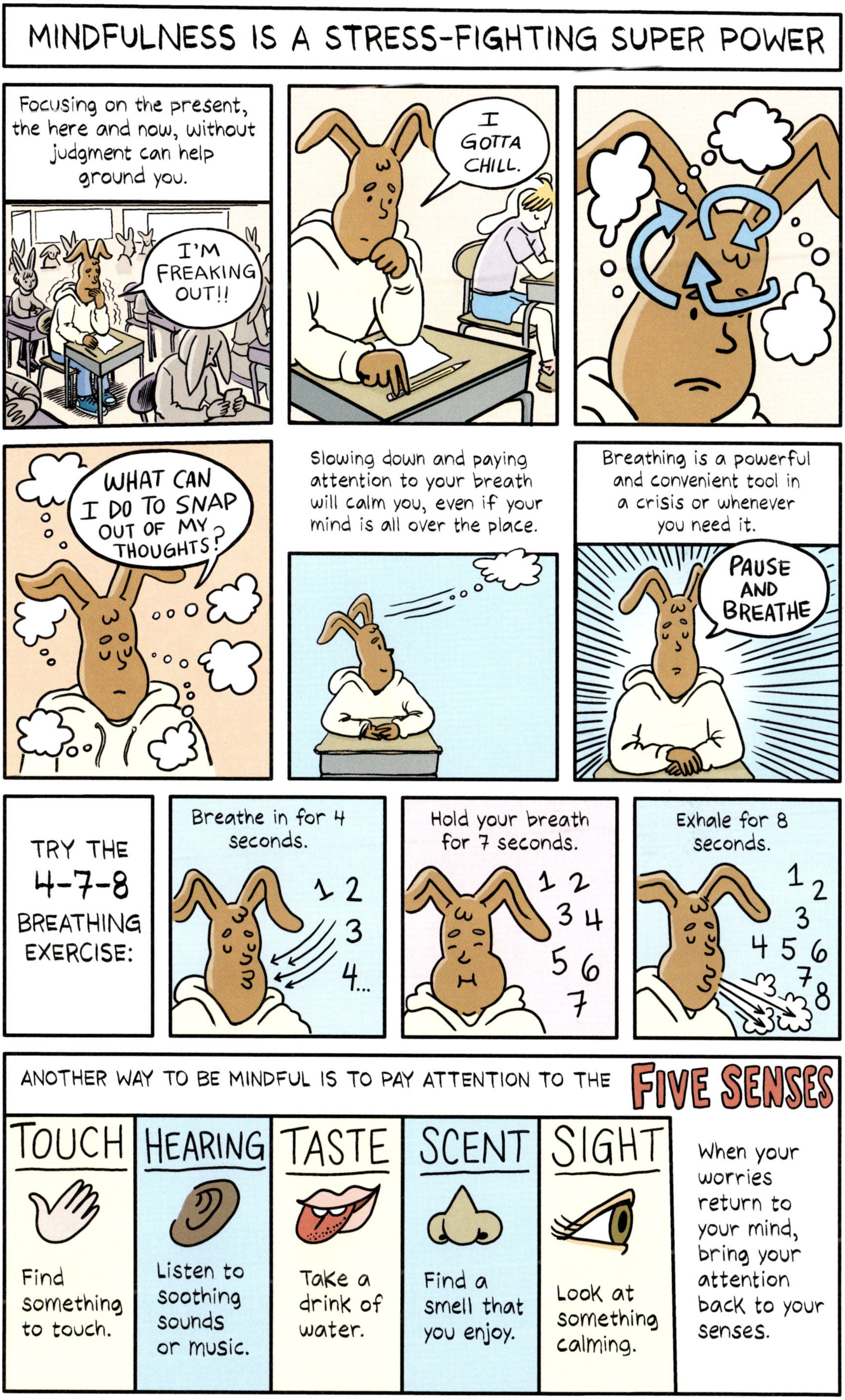

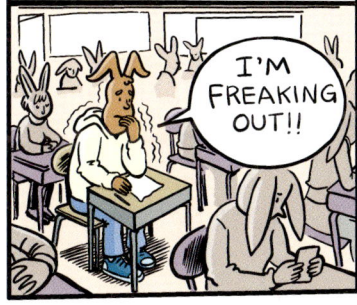

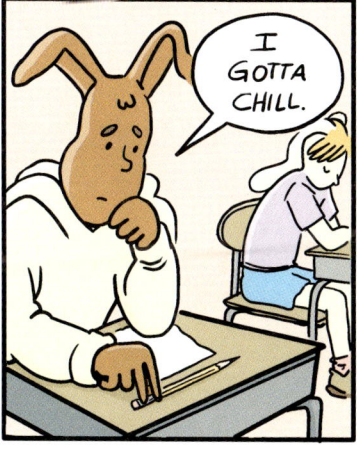

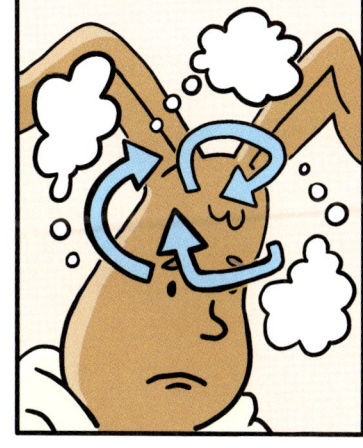

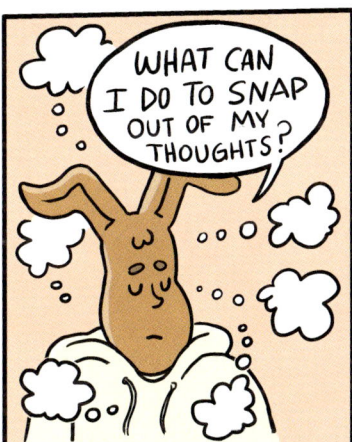

I'M FREAKING OUT!!

I GOTTA CHILL.

WHAT CAN I DO TO SNAP OUT OF MY THOUGHTS?

Slowing down and paying attention to your breath will calm you, even if your mind is all over the place.

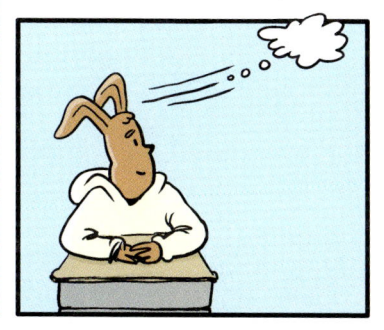

Breathing is a powerful and convenient tool in a crisis or whenever you need it.

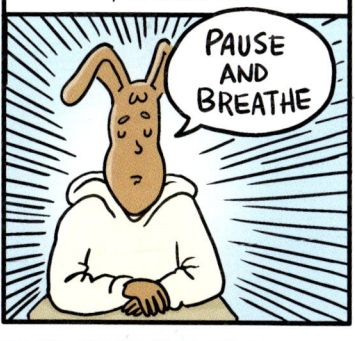

PAUSE AND BREATHE

TRY THE 4-7-8 BREATHING EXERCISE:

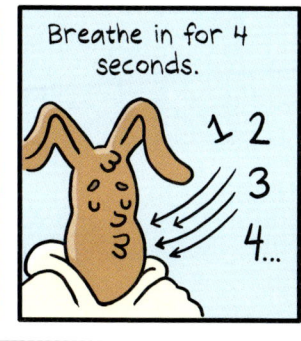

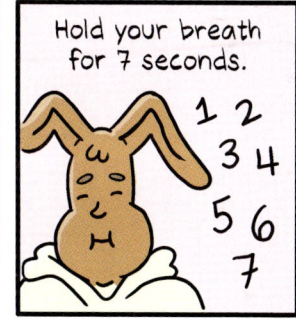

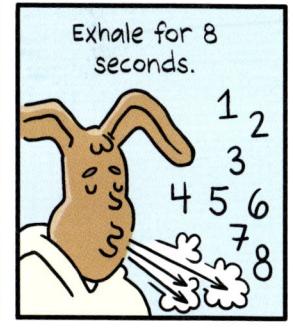

Breathe in for 4 seconds. 1 2 3 4...

Hold your breath for 7 seconds. 1 2 3 4 5 6 7

Exhale for 8 seconds. 1 2 3 4 5 6 7 8

ANOTHER WAY TO BE MINDFUL IS TO PAY ATTENTION TO THE **FIVE SENSES**

TOUCH	HEARING	TASTE	SCENT	SIGHT
Find something to touch.	Listen to soothing sounds or music.	Take a drink of water.	Find a smell that you enjoy.	Look at something calming.

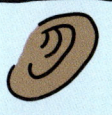

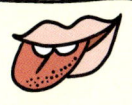

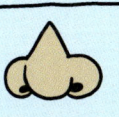

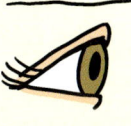

When your worries return to your mind, bring your attention back to your senses.

Mindfulness is great but sometimes...

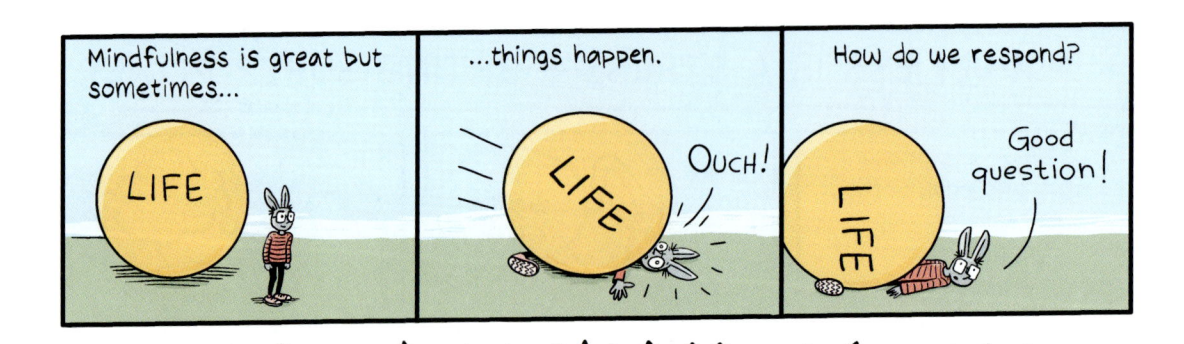

LIFE

...things happen.

LIFE Ouch!

How do we respond?

LIFE Good question!

RESILIENCE: the capacity to recover quickly from difficulties; toughness

BECOME MORE RESILIENT BY...

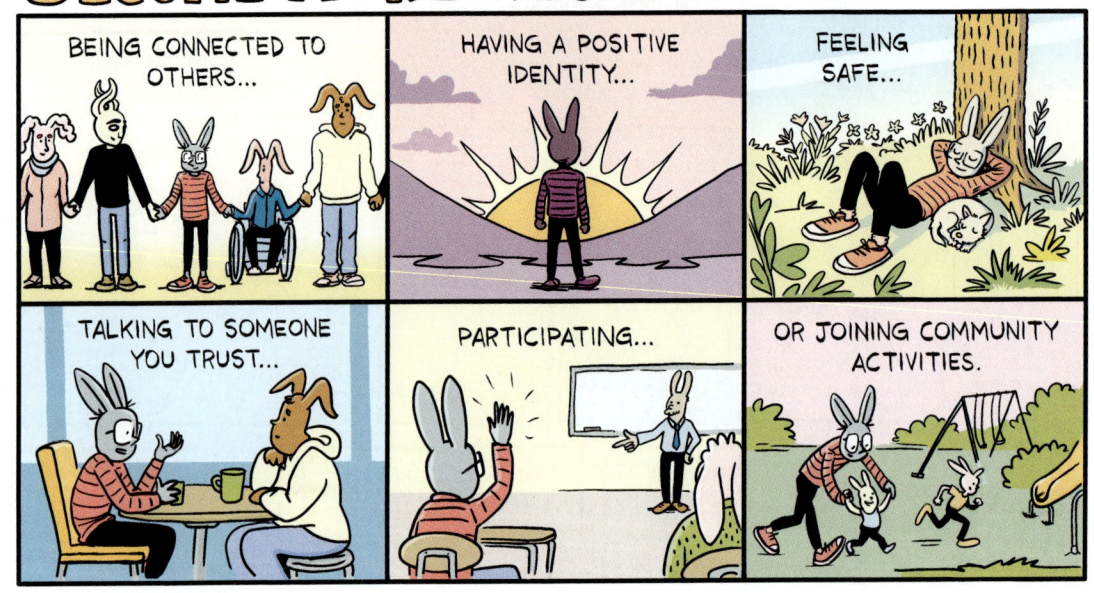

BEING CONNECTED TO OTHERS...

HAVING A POSITIVE IDENTITY...

FEELING SAFE...

TALKING TO SOMEONE YOU TRUST...

PARTICIPATING...

OR JOINING COMMUNITY ACTIVITIES.

Being part of something makes you stronger.

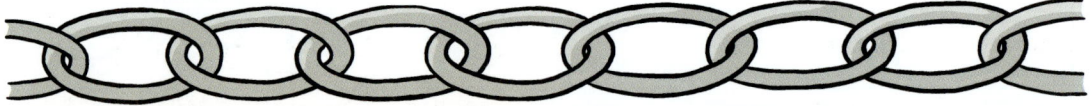

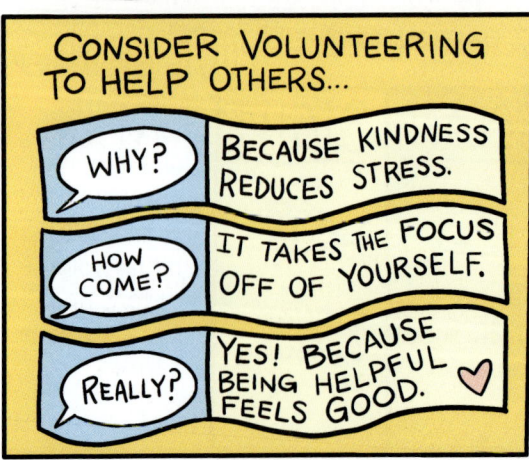

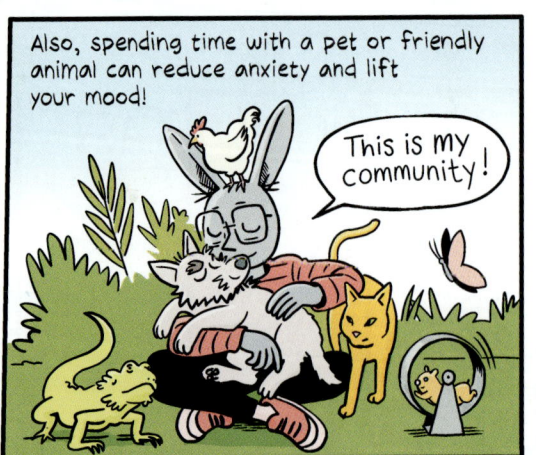

CONSIDER VOLUNTEERING TO HELP OTHERS...

WHY? BECAUSE KINDNESS REDUCES STRESS.

HOW COME? IT TAKES THE FOCUS OFF OF YOURSELF.

REALLY? YES! BECAUSE BEING HELPFUL FEELS GOOD.

Also, spending time with a pet or friendly animal can reduce anxiety and lift your mood!

This is my community!

THE PEOPLE YOU ASSOCIATE WITH INCREASE OR DECREASE YOUR RESILIENCE.	Your friend group should provide more support than drama.	"You are so cool and pretty. I feel so lucky to be your best friend."
"Don't you think it's funny that I'm your best friend, but you're not my best friend." / "Oh."	"So, I'm telling my parents that I'm sleeping over at your house this weekend. Cover for me. Okay?" / "I won't lie."	Having friends who constantly make bad choices may bring you down. / "Don't be a baby." / "I gotta go!"
Having even one good friend can help you feel better and experience less stress.	"Hi Aidy!"	"Hanging out with you is the best."

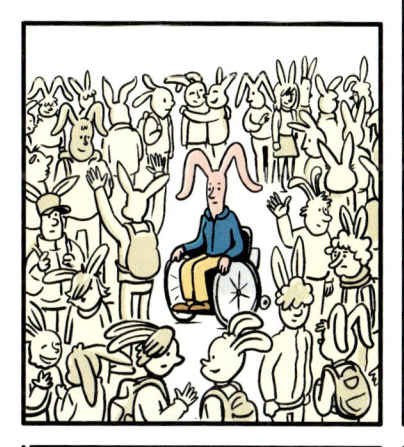

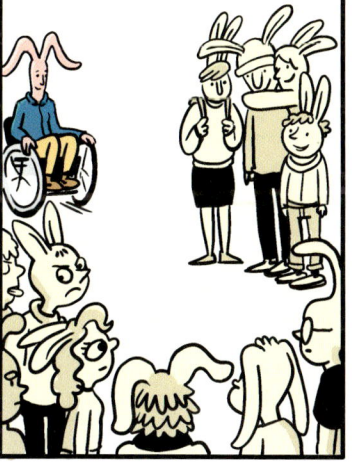

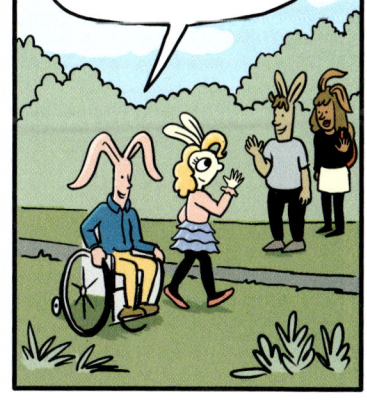

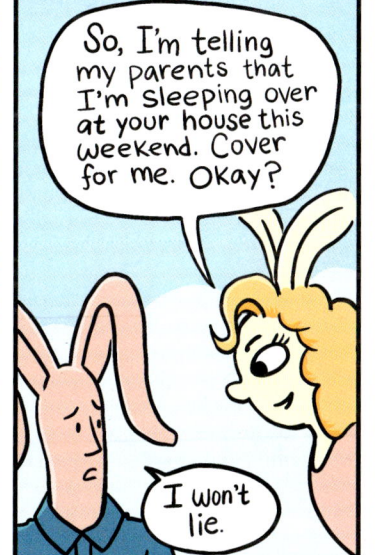

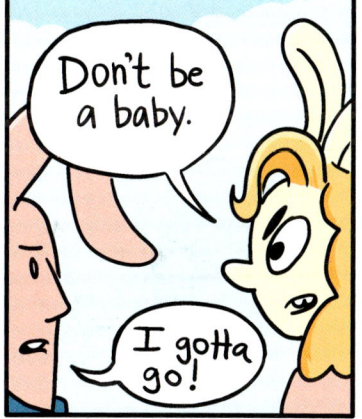

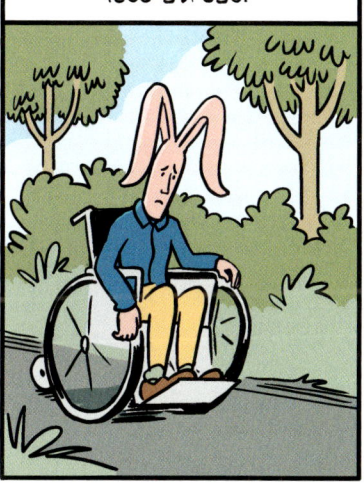

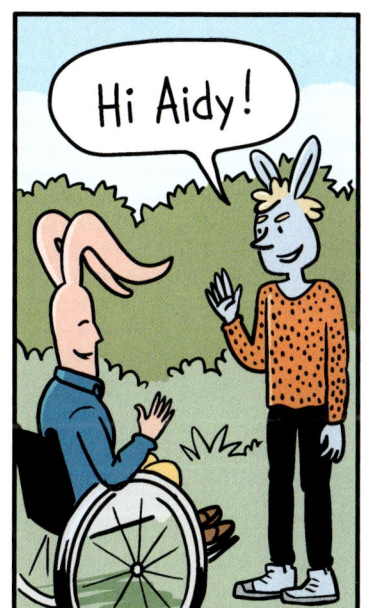

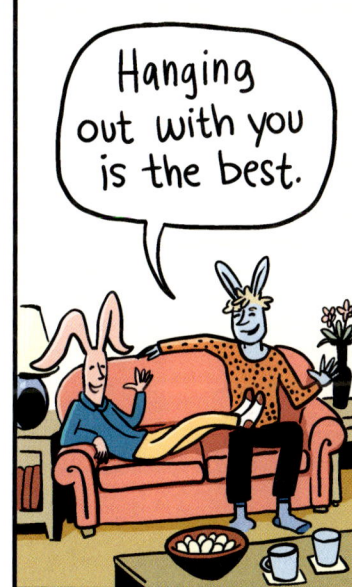

CAN A POSITIVE MINDSET IMPROVE MENTAL HEALTH?

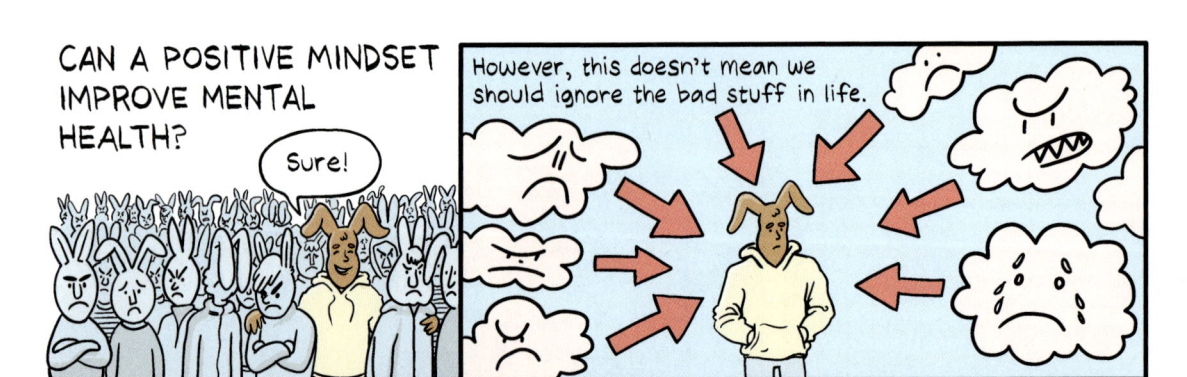

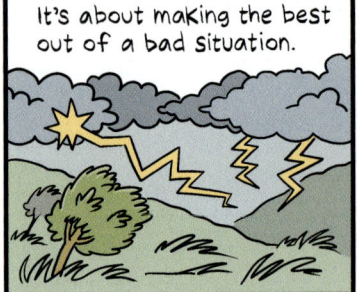

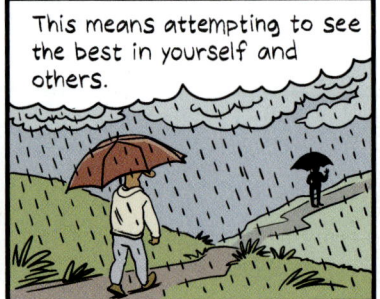

"Sure!"

However, this doesn't mean we should ignore the bad stuff in life.

It's about making the best out of a bad situation.

This means attempting to see the best in yourself and others.

Changing our mindset is a skill we can practice.

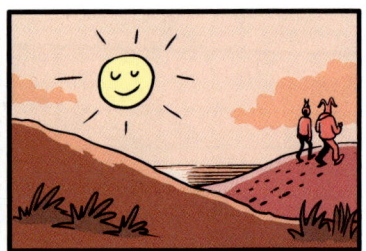

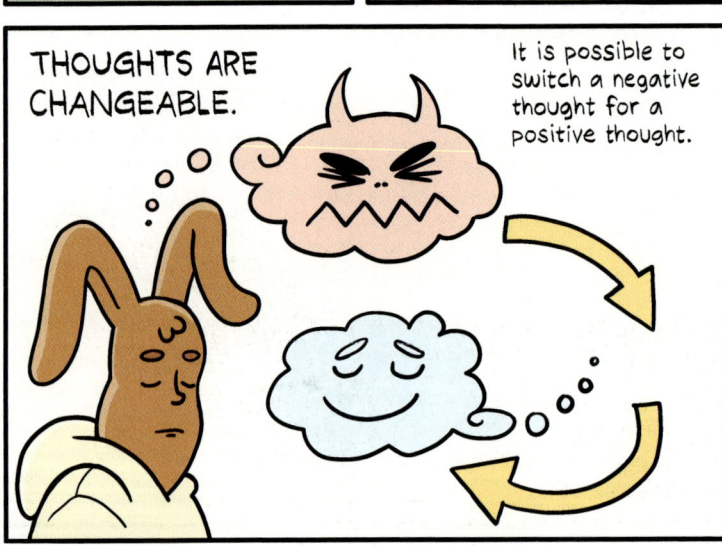

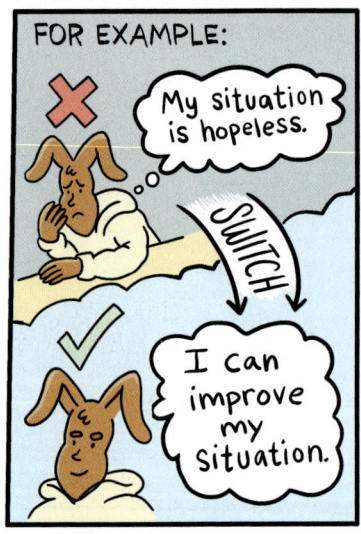

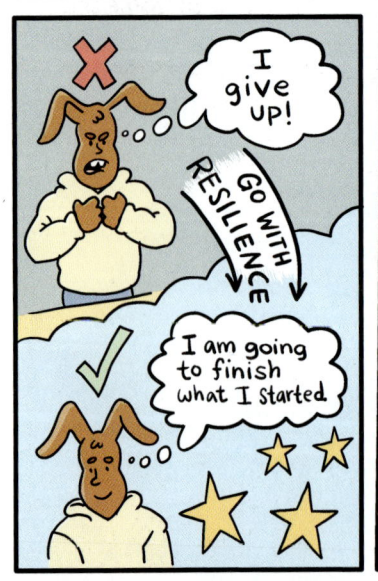

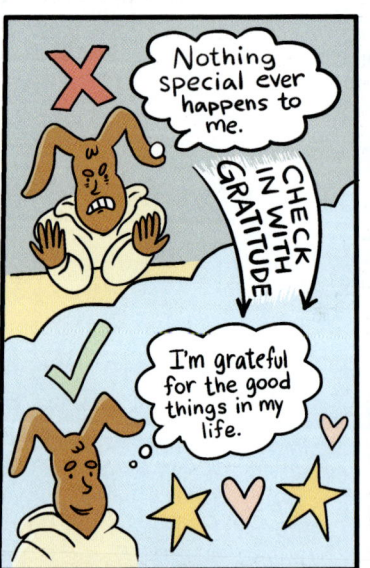

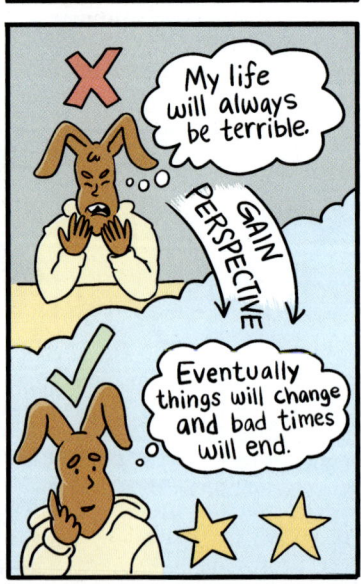

THOUGHTS ARE CHANGEABLE.

It is possible to switch a negative thought for a positive thought.

FOR EXAMPLE:

✗ "My situation is hopeless."

SWITCH

✓ "I can improve my situation."

✗ "I give up!"

GO WITH RESILIENCE

✓ "I am going to finish what I started."

✗ "Nothing special ever happens to me."

CHECK IN WITH GRATITUDE

✓ "I'm grateful for the good things in my life."

✗ "My life will always be terrible."

GAIN PERSPECTIVE

✓ "Eventually things will change and bad times will end."

There are ways that people deal with stress, painful emotions, and negative thoughts that cause harm.

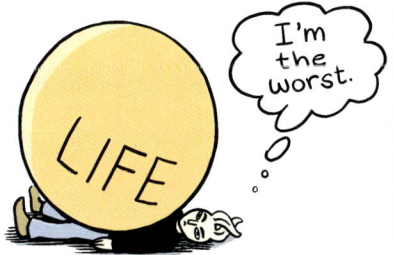

I'm the worst. — LIFE

People often keep it a secret, but the urge to harm is common.

HARM TO SOMEONE ELSE:
VIOLENCE
YELLING
BULLYING
CRUELTY

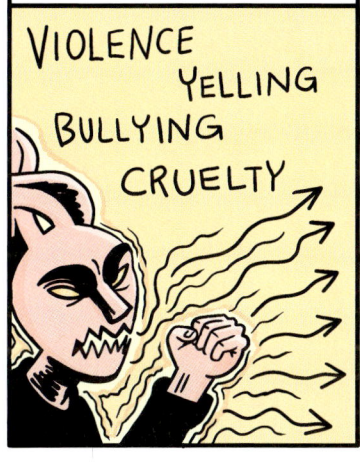

HARM TO YOURSELF:
- AVOIDANCE
- EATING DISORDER
- CUTTING, SCRATCHING, PICKING...
- DAMAGING HAIR
- DANGEROUS BEHAVIOR
- SUBSTANCE ABUSE

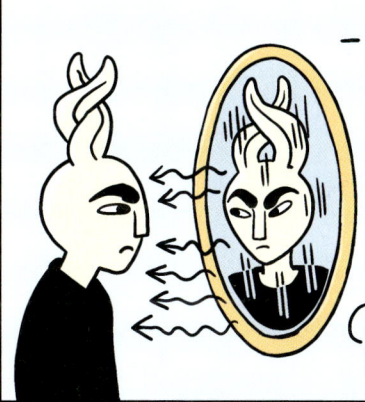

(Any behavior that hurts your body or mind.)

Acting on negative impulses can distract you from destructive feelings but it only offers temporary relief because the underlying reasons still remain.

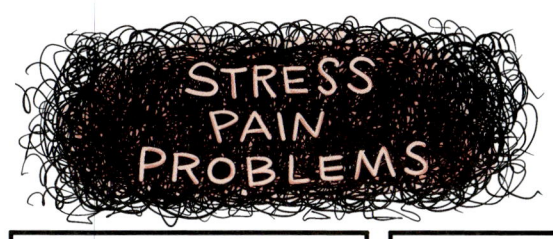

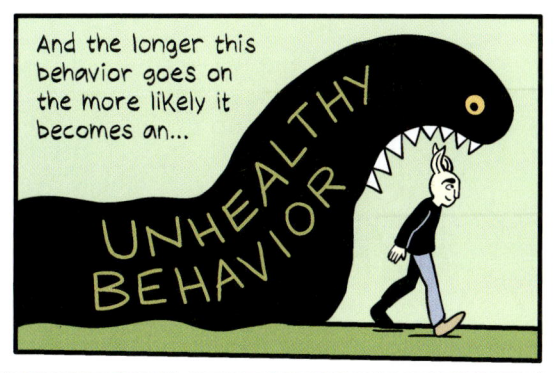

STRESS
PAIN
PROBLEMS

And the longer this behavior goes on the more likely it becomes an... UNHEALTHY BEHAVIOR

Harmful coping mechanisms can be hard to quit on your own.

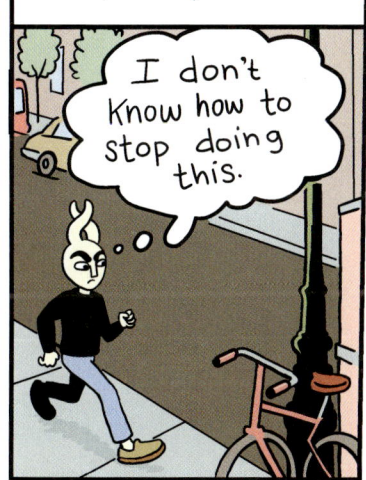

I don't know how to stop doing this.

Reaching for harmful ways to cope is a sign that there is an unmet underlying need.

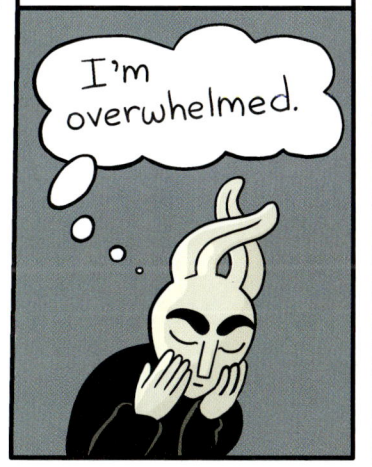

I'm overwhelmed.

Speaking to someone about it is the first step toward understanding the behavior and finding relief.

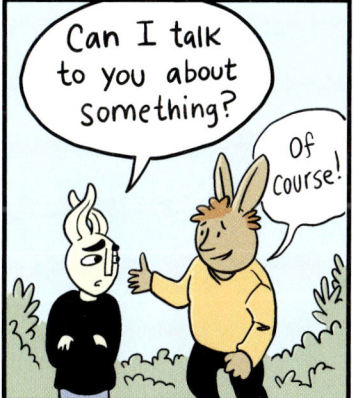

Can I talk to you about something?

Of course!

THINK ABOUT YOUR BRAIN...

...BECAUSE YOUR BRAIN IS WHAT THINKS!

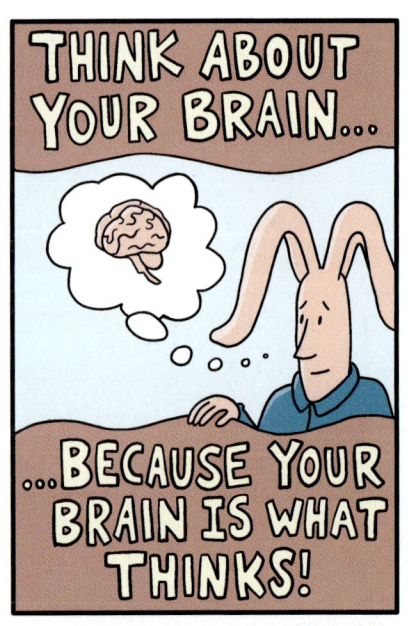

Did you know that your brain is not finished developing until you are around 25 years old?

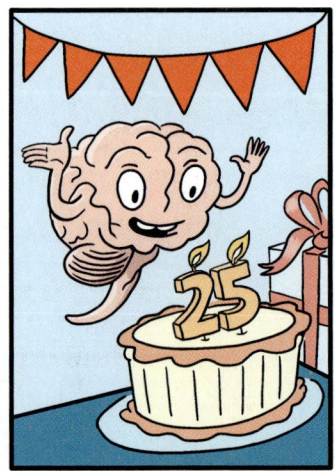

A brain goes through a dramatic change as it ages.

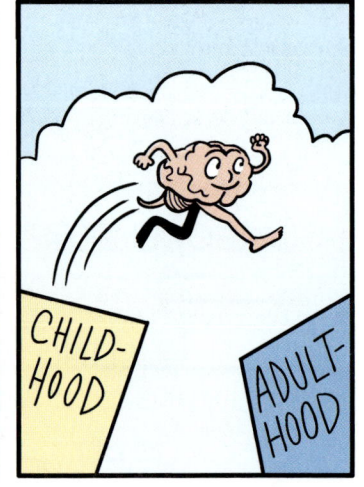

CHILDHOOD → ADULTHOOD

YOUNG BRAINS ARE VERY DIFFERENT FROM **OLD BRAINS**

"I'm fresh and new!"

"I've been around for a while."

Teen brains have more intense emotions...

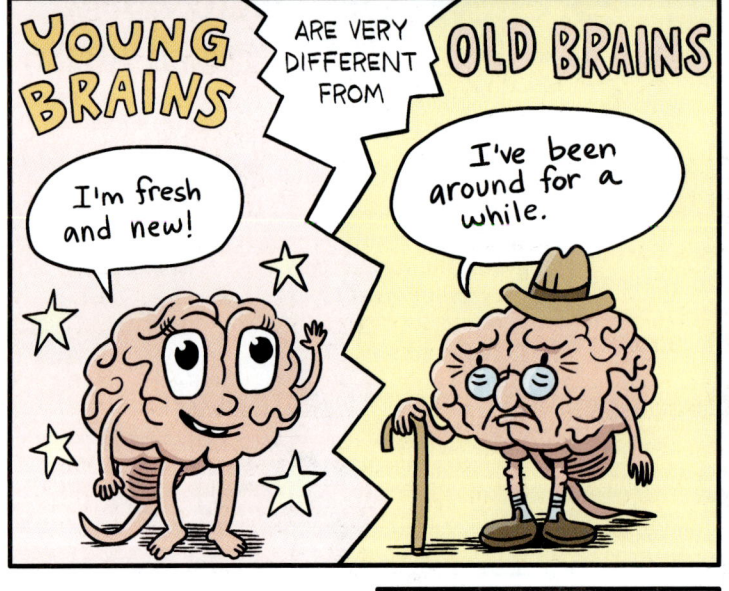

"I LOVE YOU!" "I HATE YOU!"

...and powerful learning abilities.

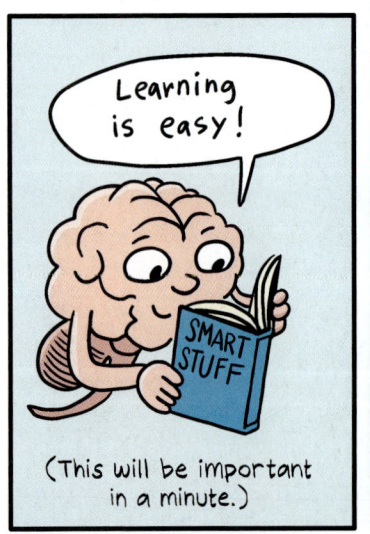

"Learning is easy!"

SMART STUFF

(This will be important in a minute.)

Adolescence also comes with intensified reward-seeking and risk-taking...

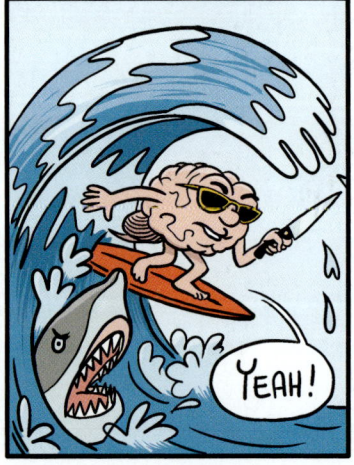

"YEAH!"

...which unfortunately can lead to substance use and addiction.

14

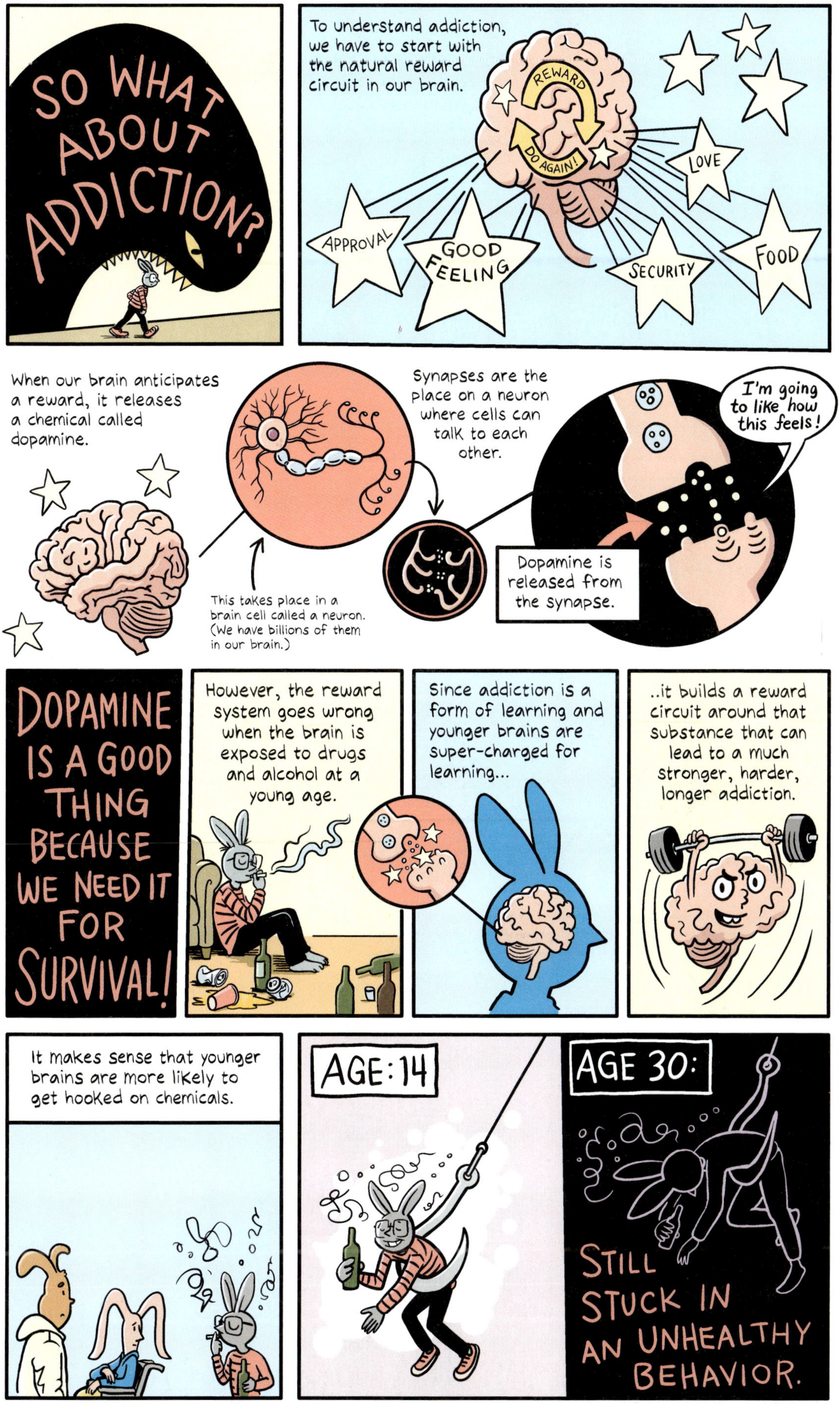

SO WHAT ABOUT ADDICTION?

To understand addiction, we have to start with the natural reward circuit in our brain.

REWARD — DO AGAIN!

APPROVAL • GOOD FEELING • LOVE • SECURITY • FOOD

When our brain anticipates a reward, it releases a chemical called dopamine.

This takes place in a brain cell called a neuron. (We have billions of them in our brain.)

Synapses are the place on a neuron where cells can talk to each other.

Dopamine is released from the synapse.

"I'm going to like how this feels!"

DOPAMINE IS A GOOD THING BECAUSE WE NEED IT FOR SURVIVAL!

However, the reward system goes wrong when the brain is exposed to drugs and alcohol at a young age.

Since addiction is a form of learning and younger brains are super-charged for learning...

...it builds a reward circuit around that substance that can lead to a much stronger, harder, longer addiction.

It makes sense that younger brains are more likely to get hooked on chemicals.

AGE: 14

AGE 30: STILL STUCK IN AN UNHEALTHY BEHAVIOR.

15

BE AWARE OF THE RISK OF SUBSTANCE USE WHILE YOUR BRAIN IS STILL DEVELOPING.

With repeated use, the chemicals in alcohol and drugs change the brain itself, making you less aware that your life is going off the rails.

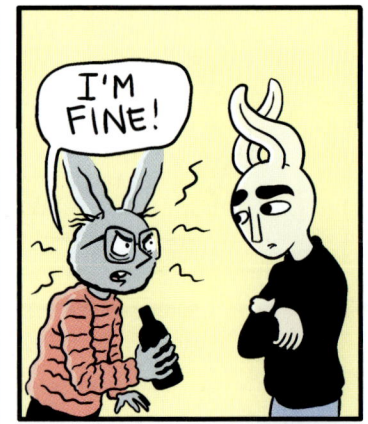

"I'M FINE!"

Things may start to go wrong at home, school, work, and in your personal life.

Repeated use also makes your life situation worse, which increases stress and feeds into the negative loop.

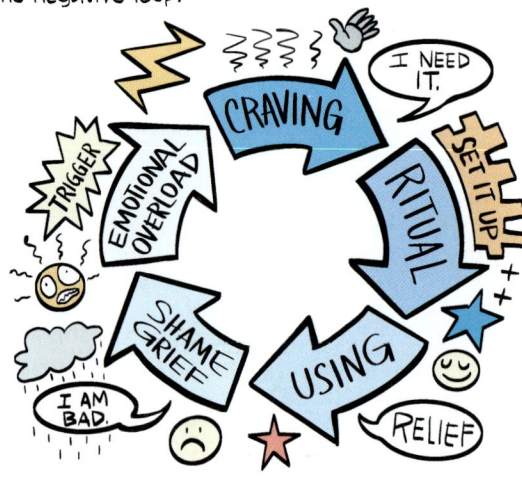

CRAVING — I NEED IT. → SET IT UP → RITUAL → USING → RELIEF → SHAME GRIEF / I AM BAD → TRIGGER → EMOTIONAL OVERLOAD → (back to CRAVING)

Without a change, addiction can lead to broken promises, damaged relationships, and tragic deaths.

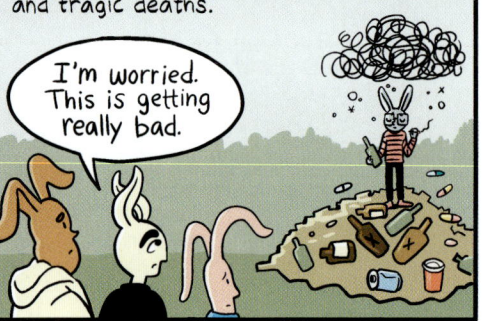

"I'm worried. This is getting really bad."

Learning to manage your emotions with healthy coping skills is better than risking brain damage.

The most reliable path for keeping your mind and body healthy and stable is to be sober by preference, choice, or necessity.

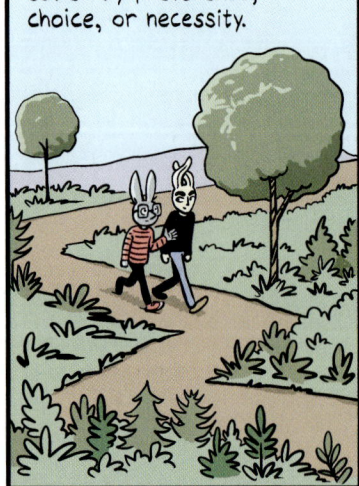

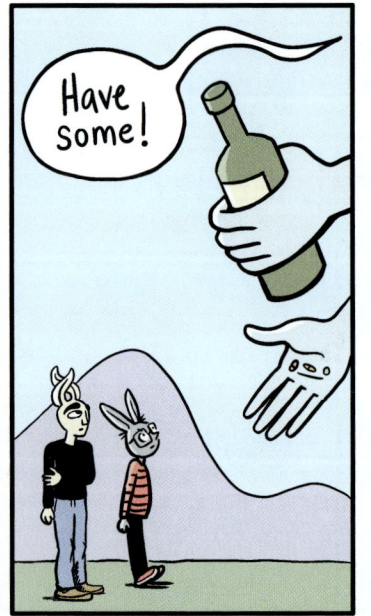

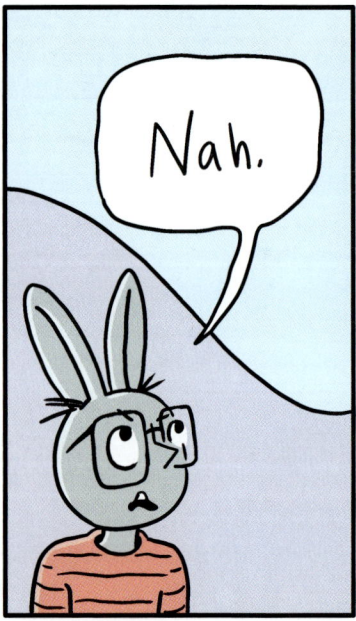

"Have some!"

"Nah."

16

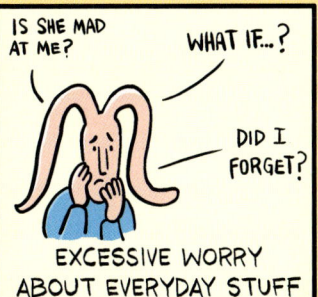

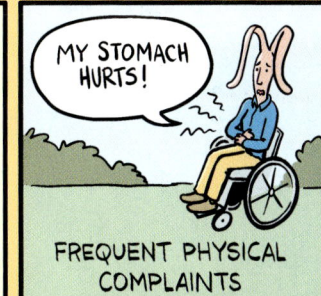

LET'S TALK ABOUT ANXIETY

Anxiety is an alarm from our brain's fight, flight or freeze response.

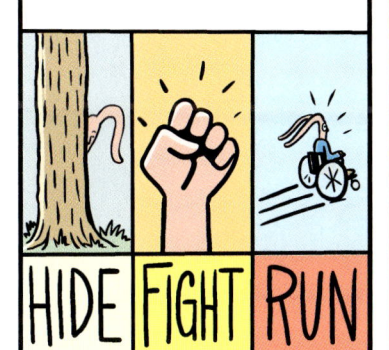

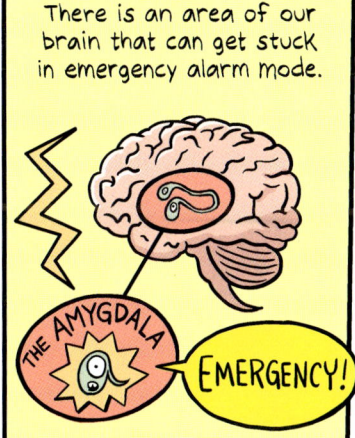

HIDE • FIGHT • RUN

There is an area of our brain that can get stuck in emergency alarm mode.

THE AMYGDALA — EMERGENCY!

Anxiety is a normal experience for all people living in this complex world. It can be a mild sensation of worry or fear...

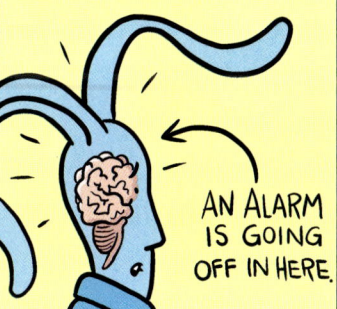

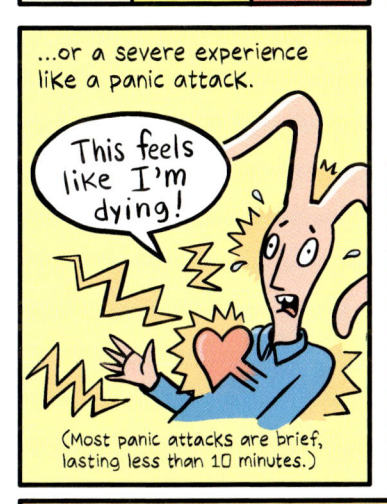

AN ALARM IS GOING OFF IN HERE.

...or a severe experience like a panic attack.

"This feels like I'm dying!"

(Most panic attacks are brief, lasting less than 10 minutes.)

There is a difference between anxiety and an anxiety disorder which does not go away on its own.

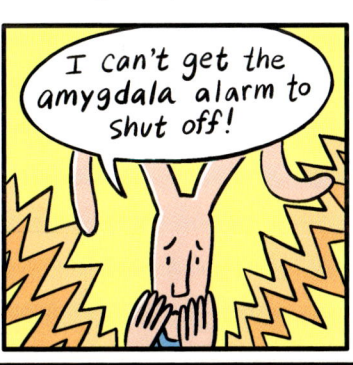

"I can't get the amygdala alarm to shut off!"

The good news is that anxiety disorders are treatable. The first step is asking for help!

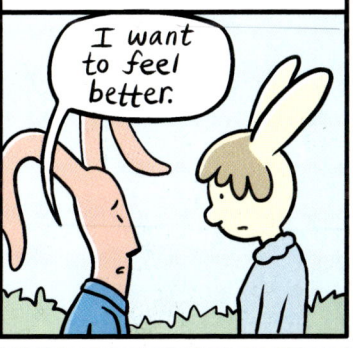

"I want to feel better."

SYMPTOMS OF ANXIETY:

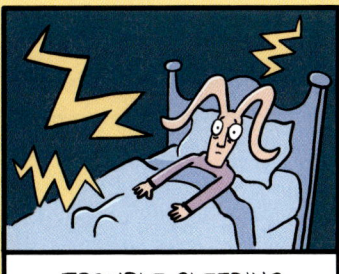

TROUBLE SLEEPING

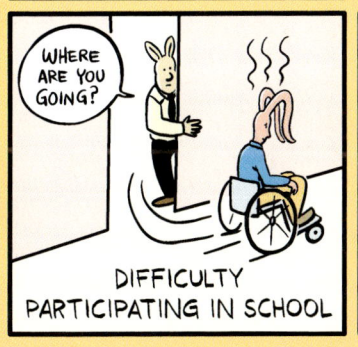

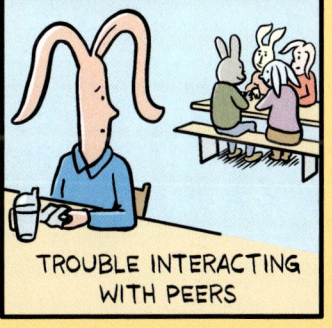

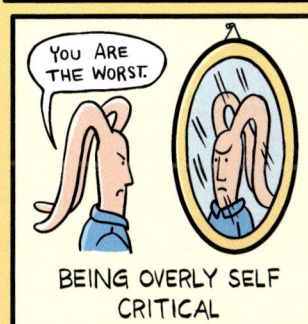

EXCESSIVE WORRY ABOUT EVERYDAY STUFF
(IS SHE MAD AT ME? WHAT IF...? DID I FORGET?)

FREQUENT PHYSICAL COMPLAINTS
"MY STOMACH HURTS!"

DIFFICULTY PARTICIPATING IN SCHOOL
"WHERE ARE YOU GOING?"

TROUBLE INTERACTING WITH PEERS

BEING OVERLY SELF CRITICAL
"YOU ARE THE WORST."

LET'S TALK ABOUT DEPRESSION

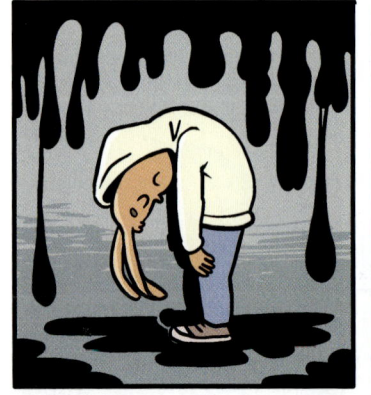

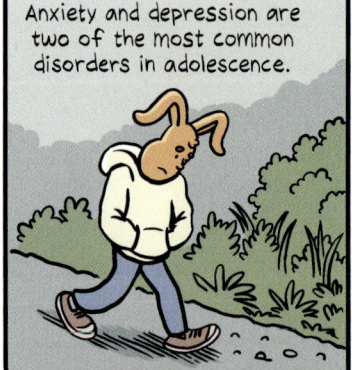

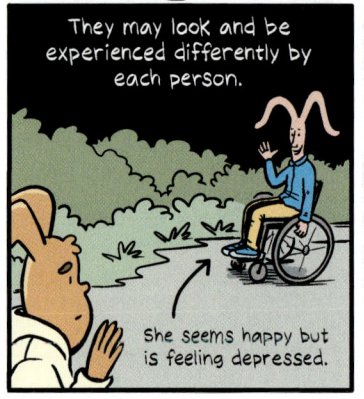

Anxiety and depression are two of the most common disorders in adolescence.

They may look and be experienced differently by each person.

She seems happy but is feeling depressed.

We know that it's normal to feel down sometimes. It's good to experience sadness and be able to talk about it.

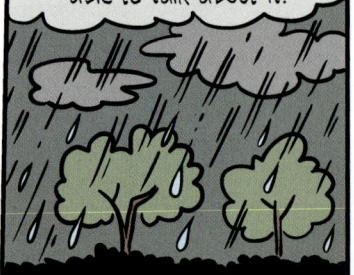

Depression is different. Depression is a disorder whose symptoms interfere with daily life and can lead to suicidal thoughts.

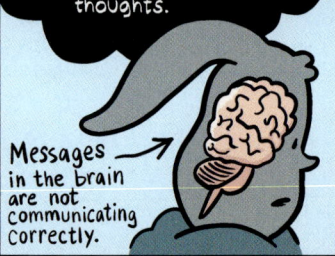

Messages in the brain are not communicating correctly.

There is help for depression! See a doctor if you experience symptoms.

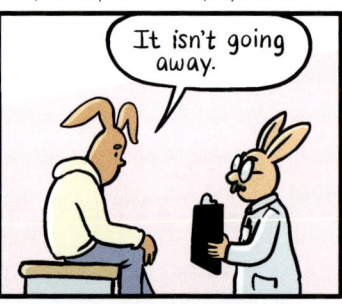

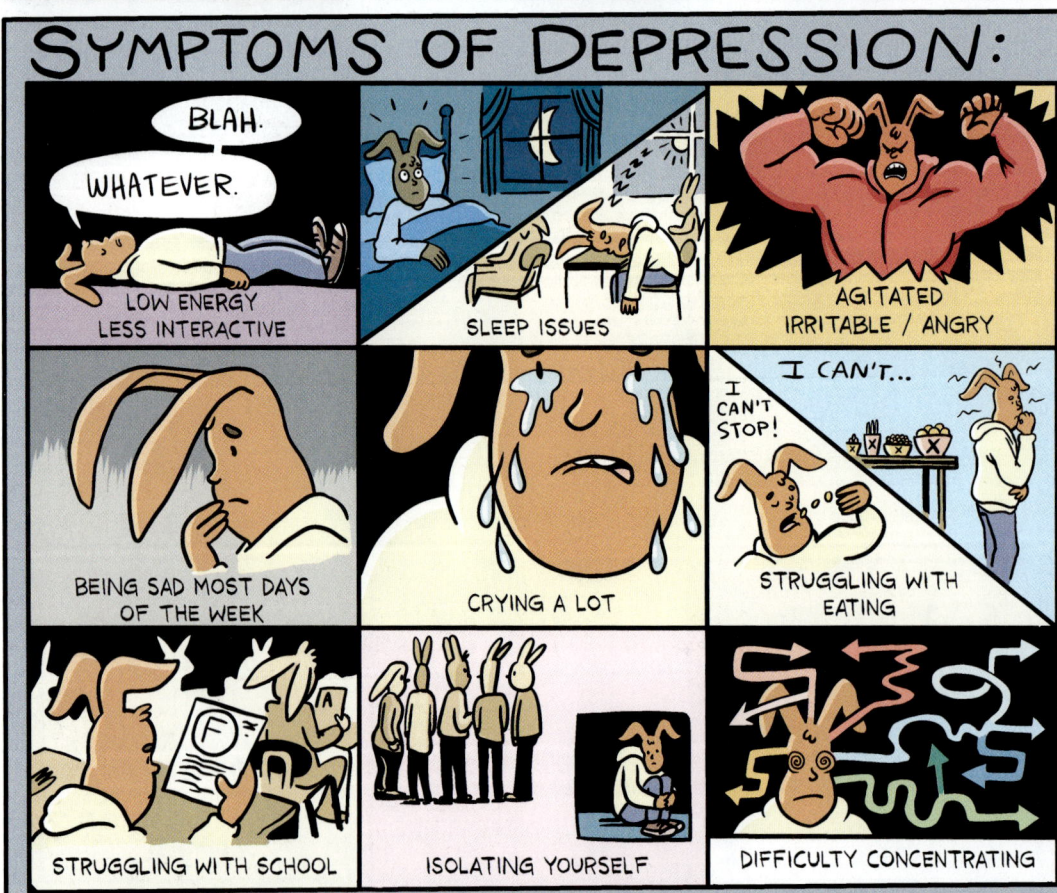

It isn't going away.

SYMPTOMS OF DEPRESSION:

BLAH. WHATEVER.
LOW ENERGY / LESS INTERACTIVE

SLEEP ISSUES

AGITATED / IRRITABLE / ANGRY

BEING SAD MOST DAYS OF THE WEEK

CRYING A LOT

I CAN'T STOP! **I CAN'T...**
STRUGGLING WITH EATING

STRUGGLING WITH SCHOOL

ISOLATING YOURSELF

DIFFICULTY CONCENTRATING

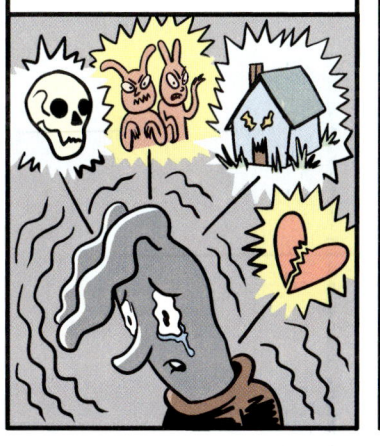

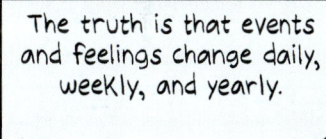

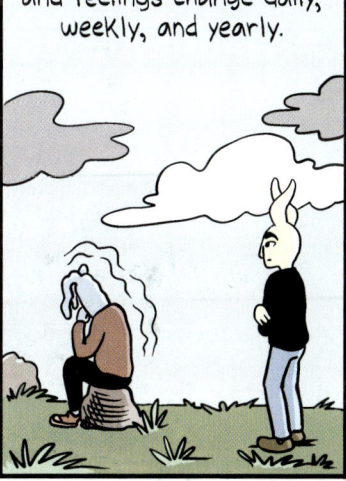

Addressing Thoughts About Suicide

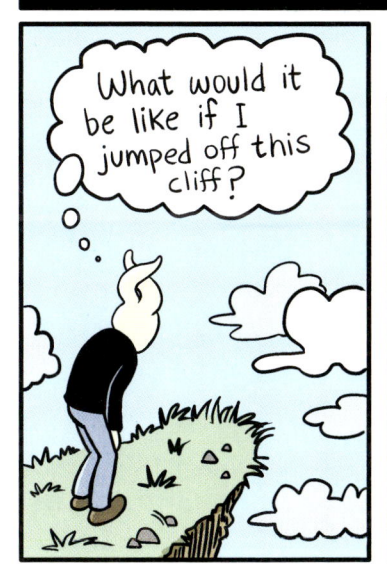

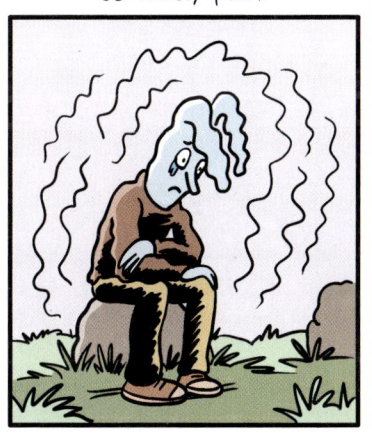

What would it be like if I jumped off this cliff?

Everybody thinks about it a little bit.

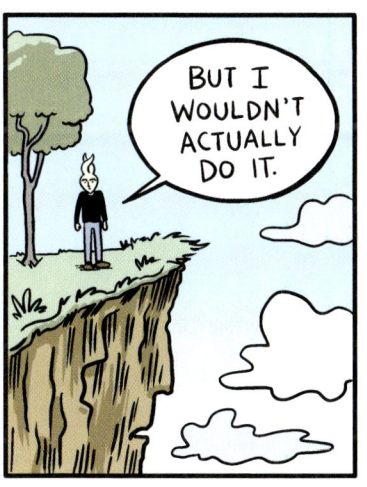

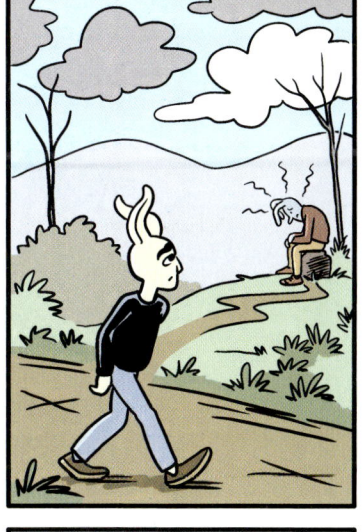

BUT I WOULDN'T ACTUALLY DO IT.

For some people, suicide is something they may actually begin to seriously plan.

It can seem like the stress is too much to handle.

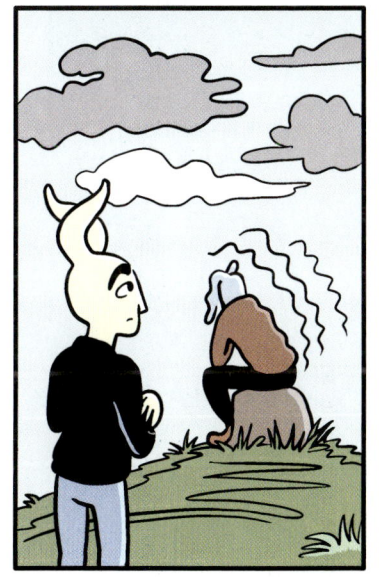

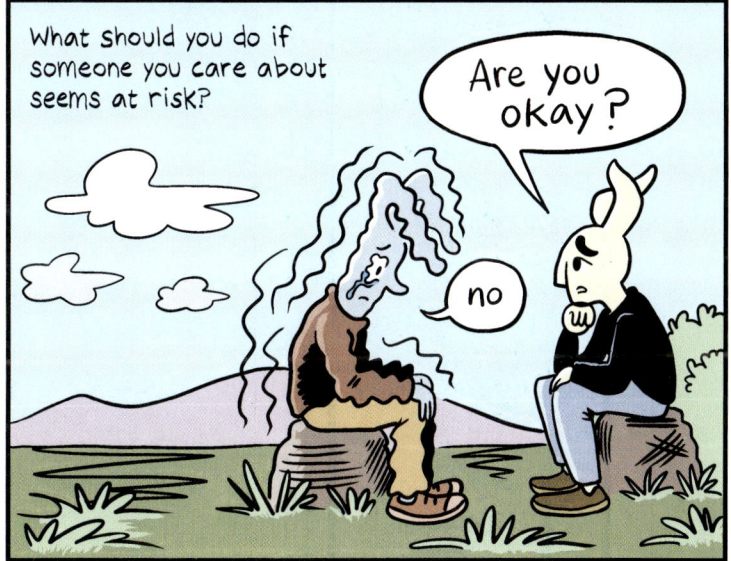

The truth is that events and feelings change daily, weekly, and yearly.

What should you do if someone you care about seems at risk?

Are you okay?

no

A Conversation About Suicide

You might be the person someone reaches out to in a crisis.

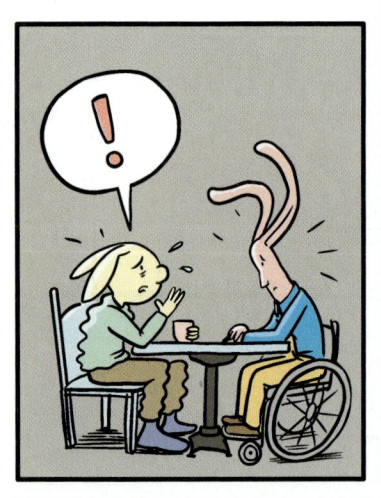

Know that talking about suicide does not cause someone to be suicidal.

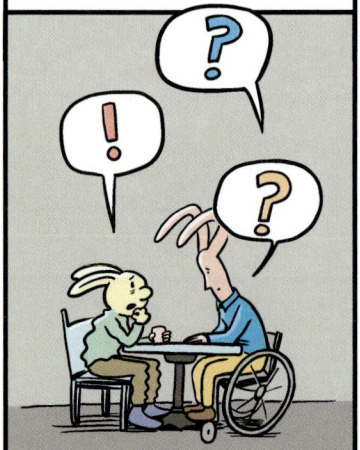

Don't keep secrets about suicide. Talk to a trusted adult if you are worried about your friend.

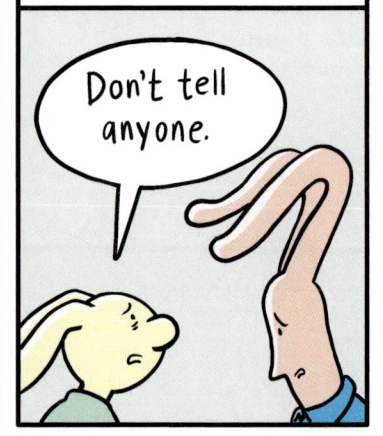

"Don't tell anyone."

It is better to lose a friendship than a friend.

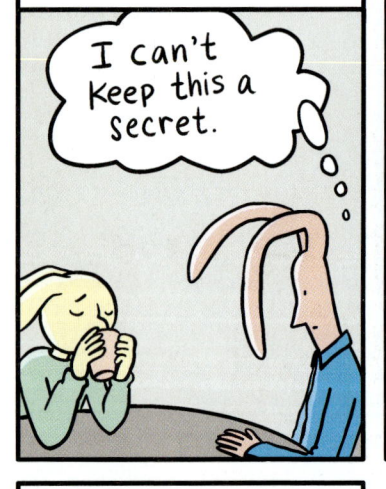

"I can't keep this a secret."

Most people want to live; they are just unable to see alternatives to their problems.

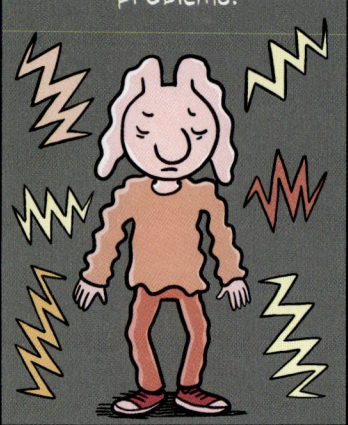

It's okay to ask directly.

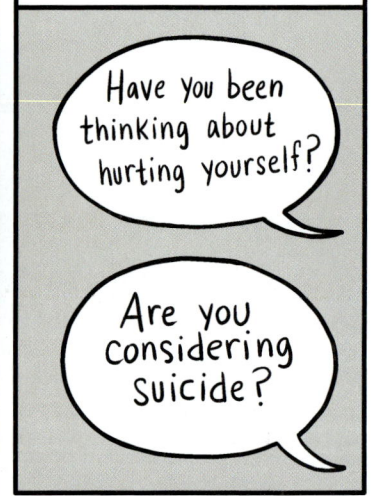

"Have you been thinking about hurting yourself?"

"Are you considering suicide?"

Remember that if you have immediate concerns, you can call 911 right away.

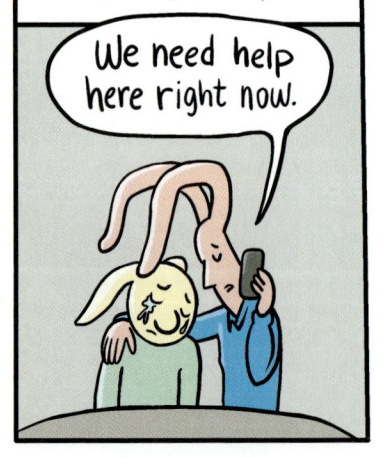

"We need help here right now."

You can encourage your friend to call or text the National Suicide Prevention Lifeline at:

988

By taking the time to notice and reach out to a peer, you can be at the beginning of a positive solution.

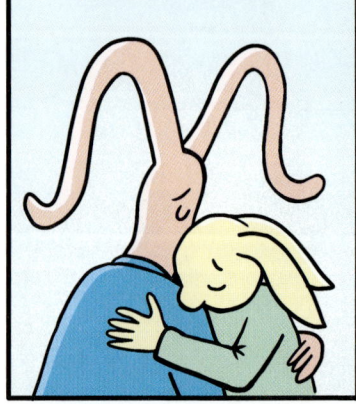

There is help out there for you no matter what you're struggling with.

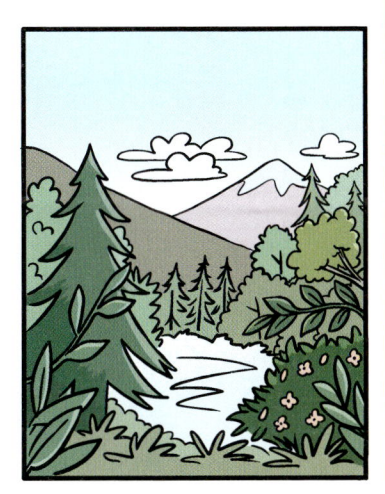

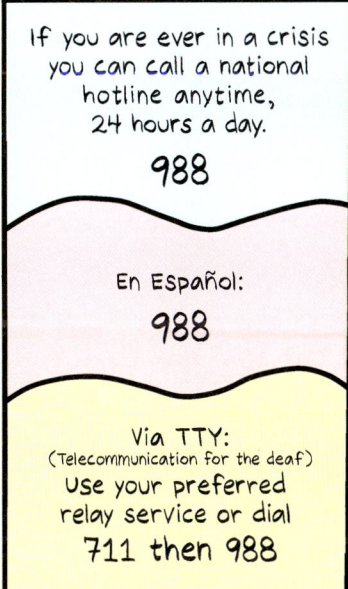

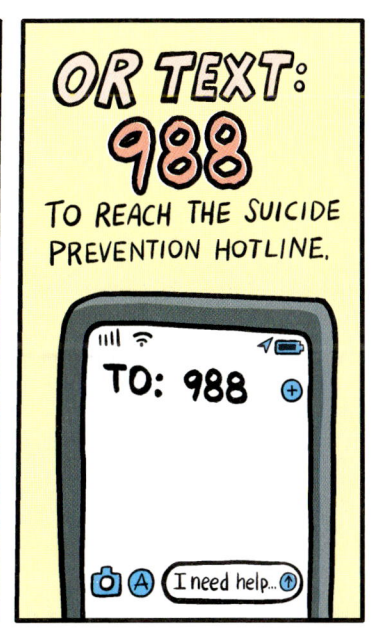

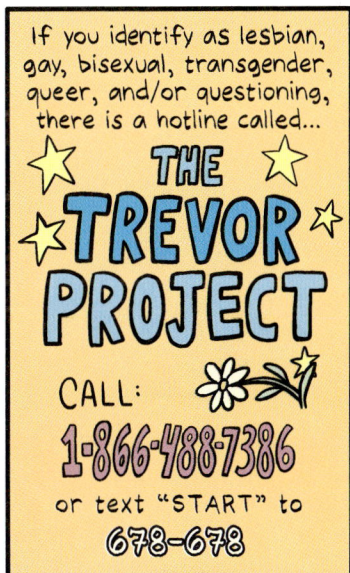

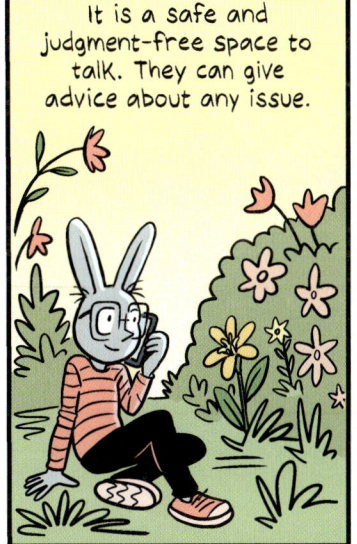

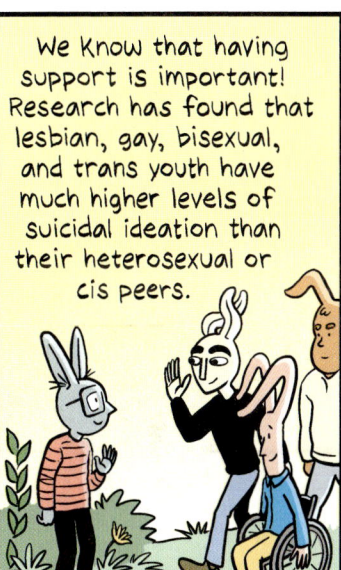

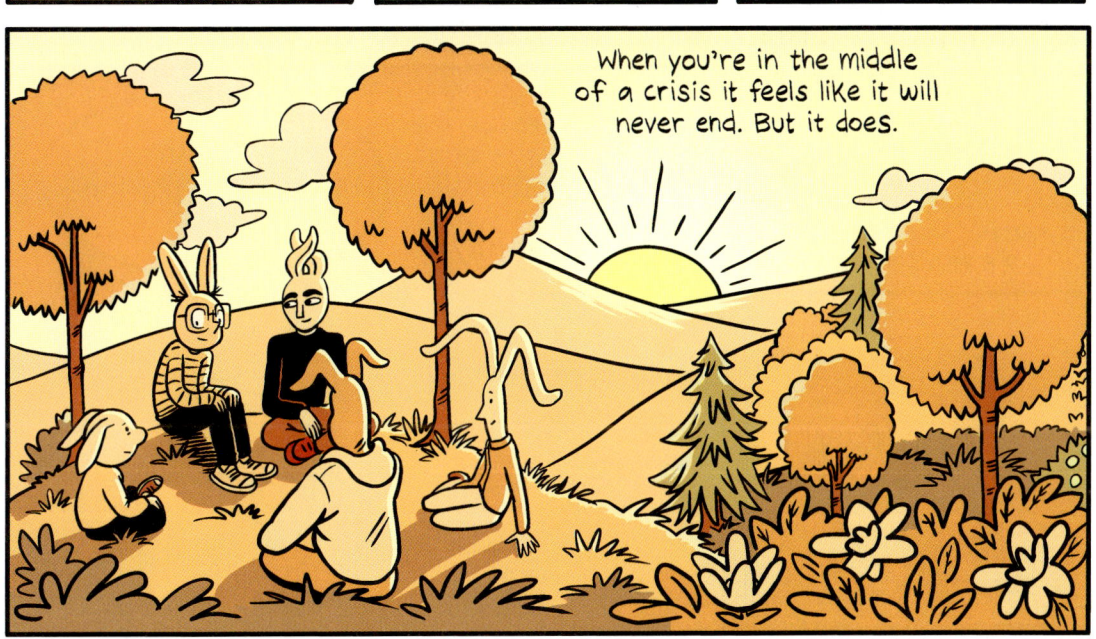

If you are ever in a crisis you can call a national hotline anytime, 24 hours a day.

988

En Español:
988

Via TTY:
(Telecommunication for the deaf)
Use your preferred relay service or dial
711 then 988

OR TEXT:
988
TO REACH THE SUICIDE PREVENTION HOTLINE.

TO: 988

I need help...

If you identify as lesbian, gay, bisexual, transgender, queer, and/or questioning, there is a hotline called...

THE TREVOR PROJECT

CALL:
1-866-488-7386
or text "START" to
678-678

It is a safe and judgment-free space to talk. They can give advice about any issue.

We know that having support is important! Research has found that lesbian, gay, bisexual, and trans youth have much higher levels of suicidal ideation than their heterosexual or cis peers.

When you're in the middle of a crisis it feels like it will never end. But it does.

21

Seek Help For Your Mental Health

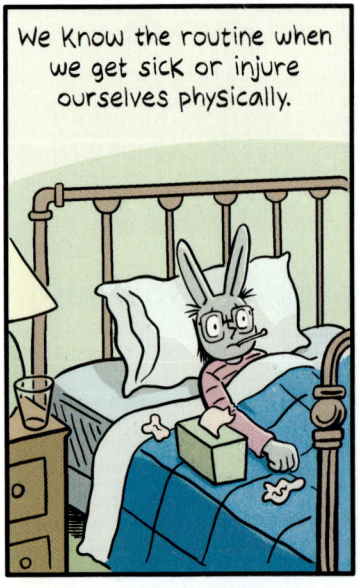

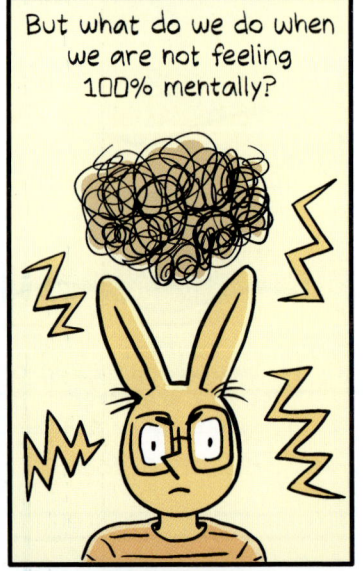

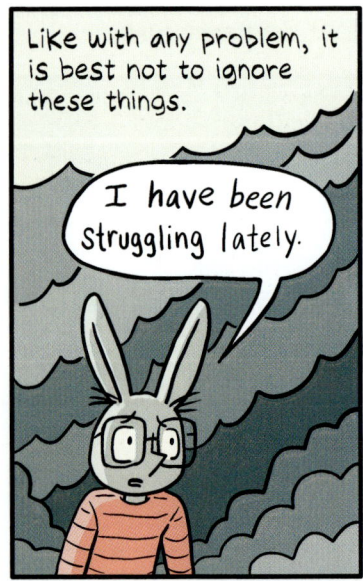

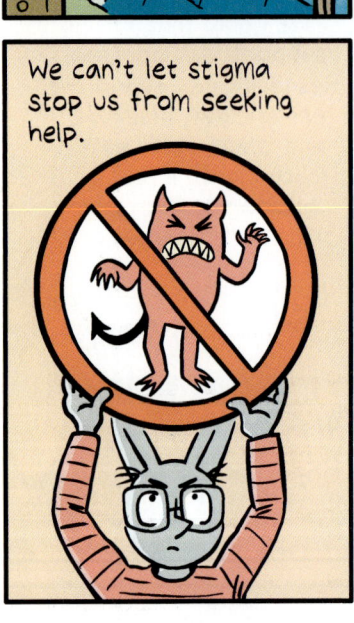

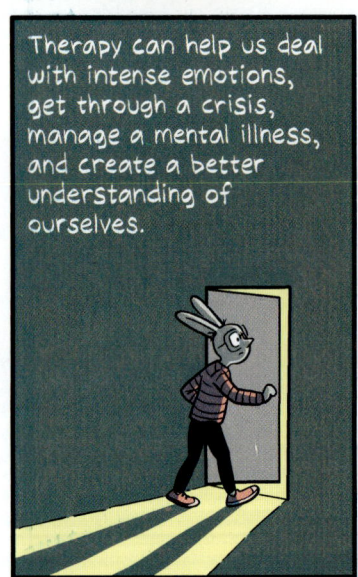

We know the routine when we get sick or injure ourselves physically.

But what do we do when we are not feeling 100% mentally?

Like with any problem, it is best not to ignore these things.

"I have been struggling lately."

We can't let stigma stop us from seeking help.

Therapy can help us deal with intense emotions, get through a crisis, manage a mental illness, and create a better understanding of ourselves.

If you or your family are concerned about how to pay for mental health or substance use services, don't let that stop you from seeking help.

Talk to your local mental health/substance use board about options to help pay for services.

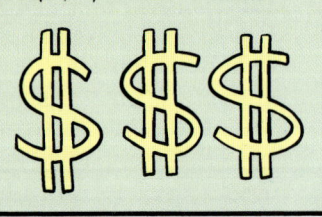

To begin, seek help from a trusted adult at home, school, etc., who can help you. Next, visit a doctor for a medical exam to check whether your symptoms could be related to a physical illness.

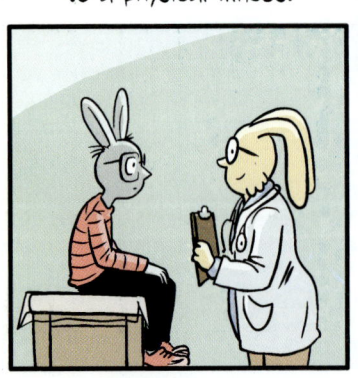

After medical disorders have been ruled out, then it's time to get referred to a mental health professional.

"This is an urgent situation."

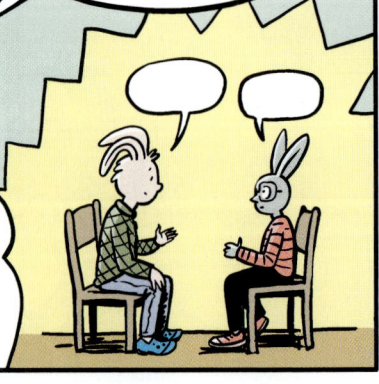

Keep in mind that it can take a while to get an appointment with a specialist. If you need to see a specialist right away, speak up to get an appointment sooner.

How to Start Seeing a Therapist

In the beginning you may be asked to complete a questionnaire or answer a series of questions.

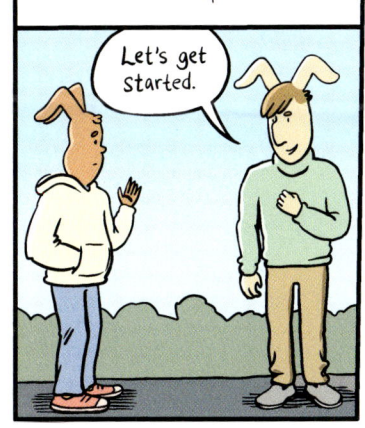

"Let's get started."

Be ready to talk about your health history and what you're experiencing.

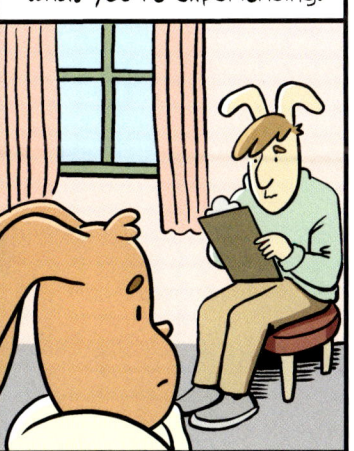

Feel free to ask questions about what will happen in your treatment.

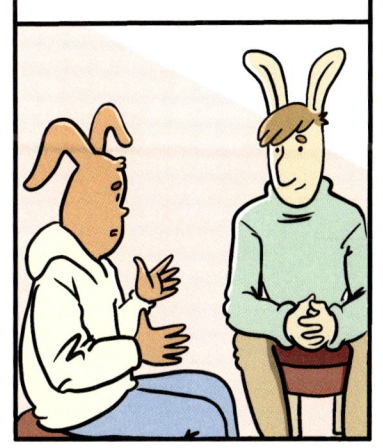

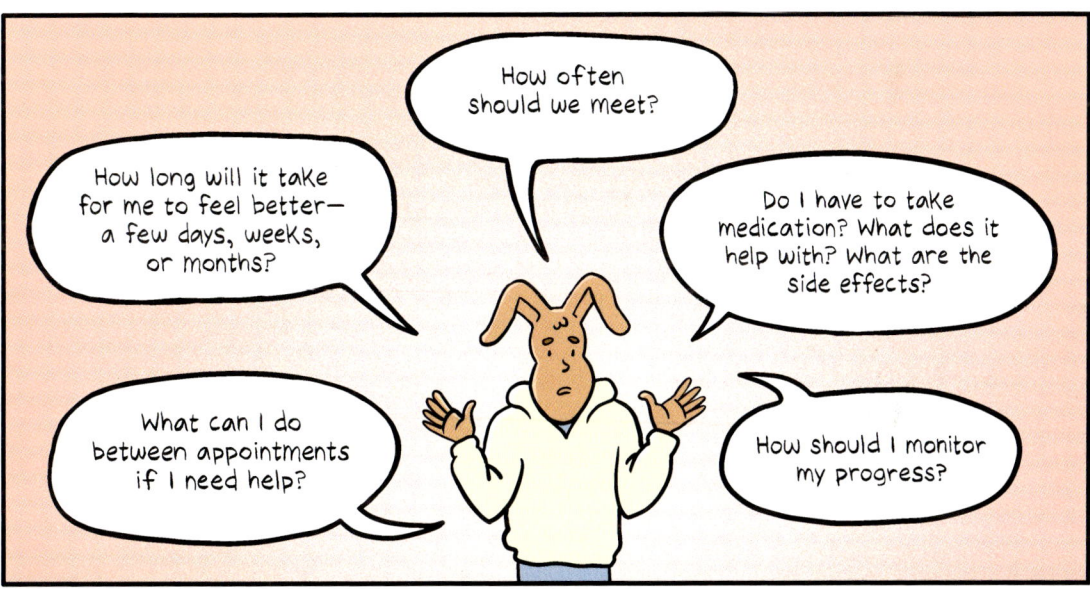

How long will it take for me to feel better—a few days, weeks, or months?

How often should we meet?

Do I have to take medication? What does it help with? What are the side effects?

What can I do between appointments if I need help?

How should I monitor my progress?

The goal is to connect with an adult in the field of psychology that you trust and can talk to.

It's good to have someone you feel safe with who really listens.

Research shows again and again that the most important factor in positive therapy outcomes is the RELATIONSHIP between the therapist and client.

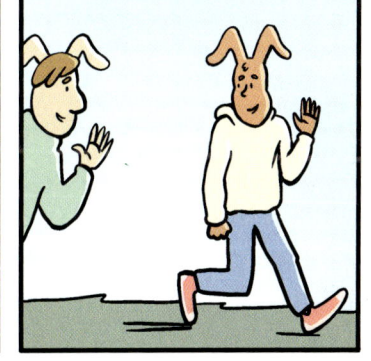

IT IS OKAY TO HAVE A MENTAL HEALTH DISORDER

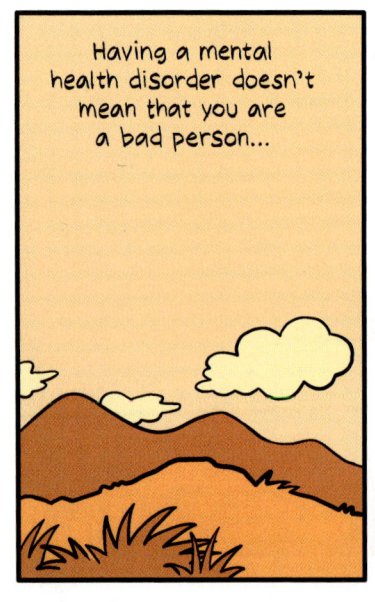

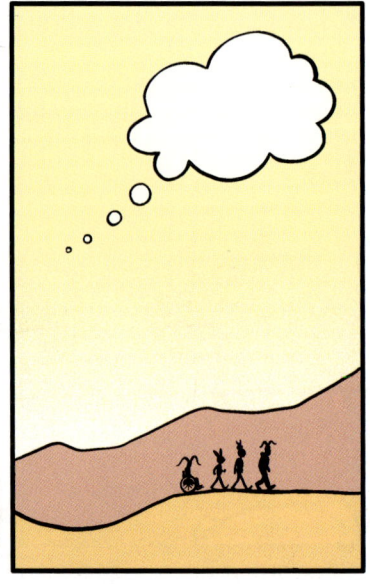

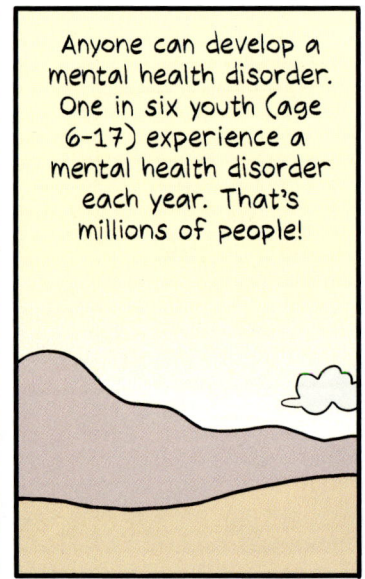

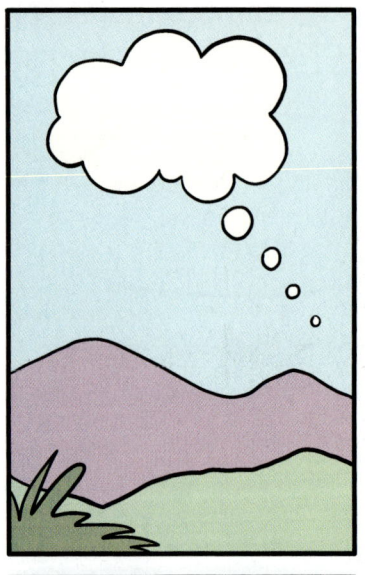

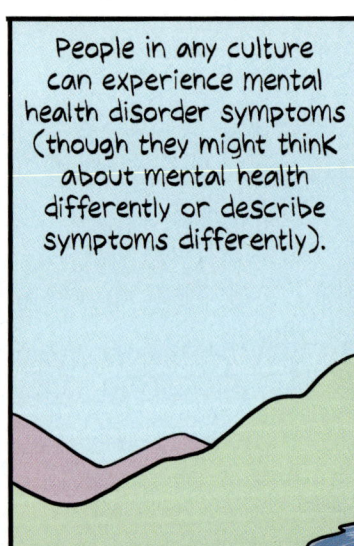

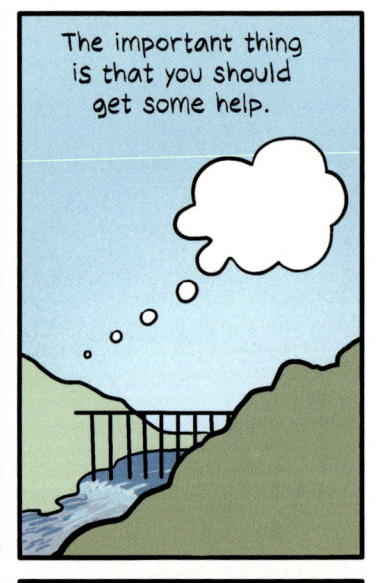

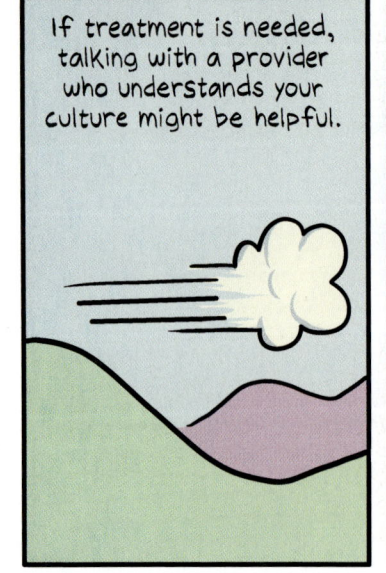

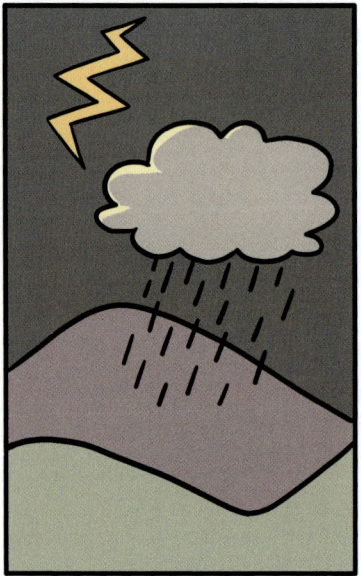

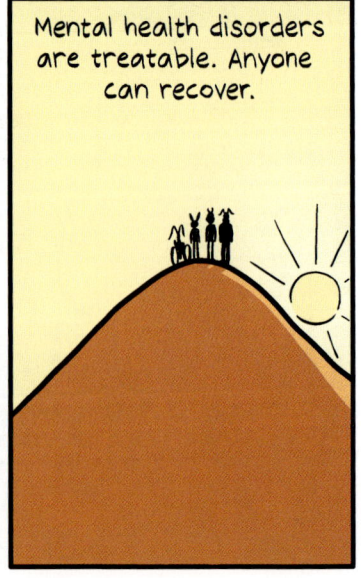

Having a mental health disorder doesn't mean that you are a bad person...

Anyone can develop a mental health disorder. One in six youth (age 6-17) experience a mental health disorder each year. That's millions of people!

People in any culture can experience mental health disorder symptoms (though they might think about mental health differently or describe symptoms differently).

The important thing is that you should get some help.

If treatment is needed, talking with a provider who understands your culture might be helpful.

Mental health disorders are treatable. Anyone can recover.

Mental Health Resources

There are many kinds of therapies and organizations that support mental health.

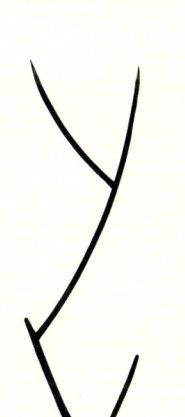

Each person's situation and experience is unique.

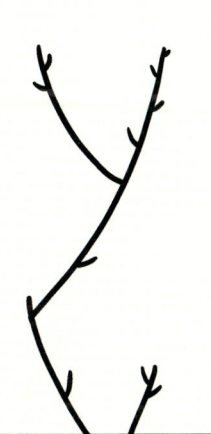

The important thing is to find the resources that work best for you.

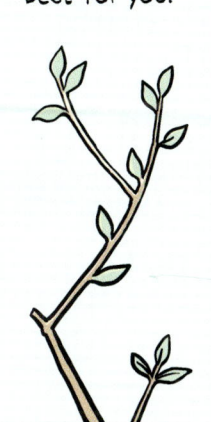

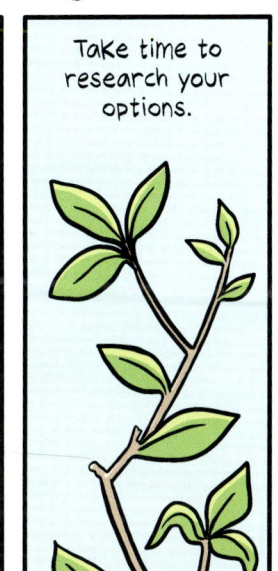

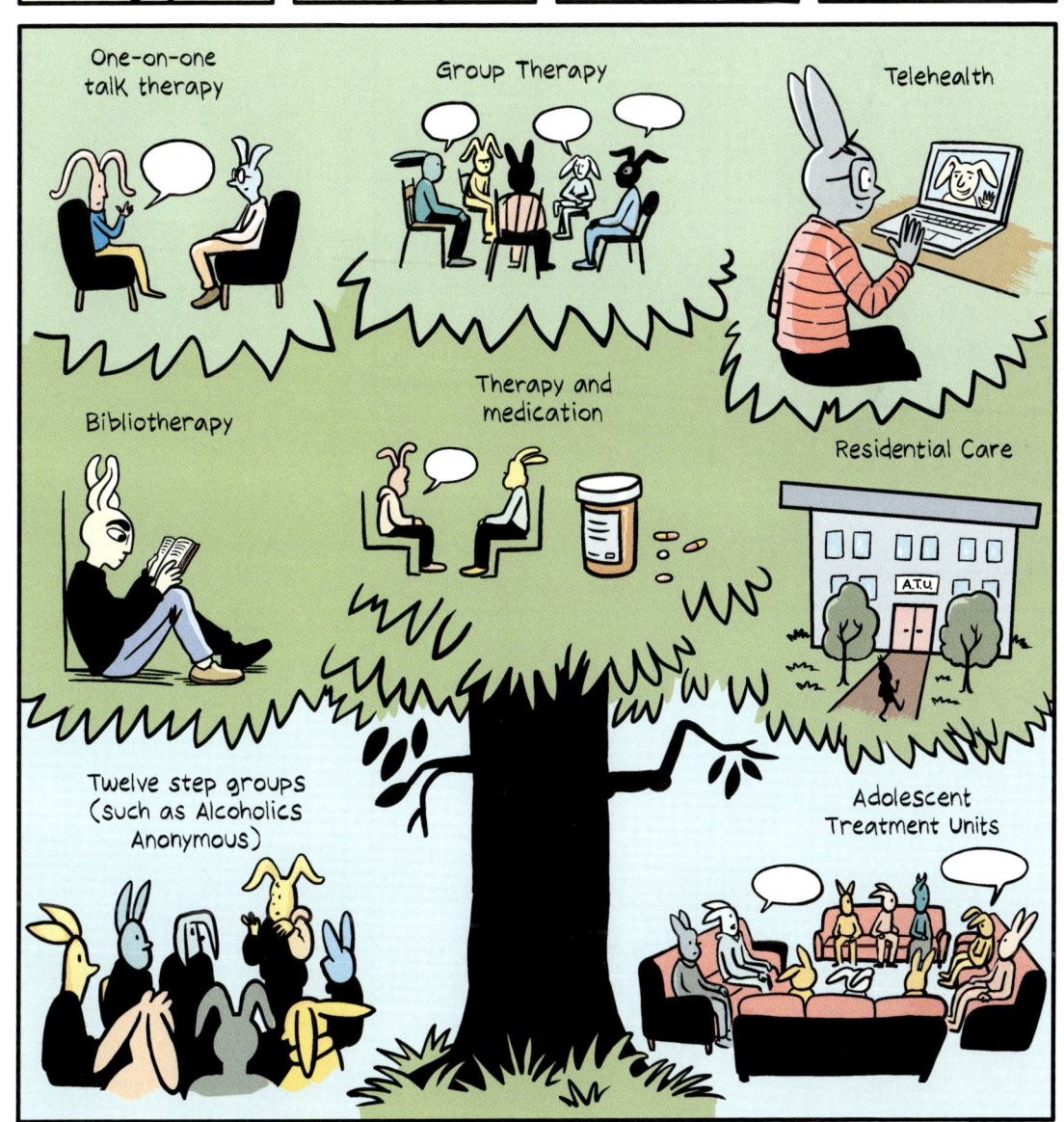

Take time to research your options.

One-on-one talk therapy

Group Therapy

Telehealth

Bibliotherapy

Therapy and medication

Residential Care

Twelve step groups (such as Alcoholics Anonymous)

Adolescent Treatment Units

TO THOSE WHO WANT TO TALK ABOUT IT...
There are many ways to start a conversation about or advocate for mental health.

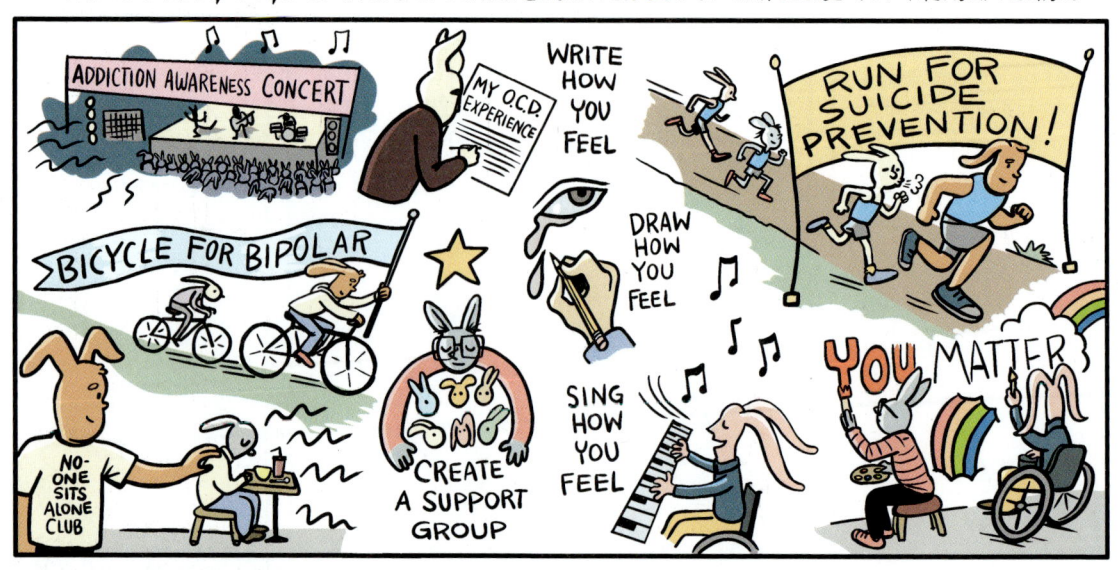

TO THOSE WHO ARE SUFFERING...

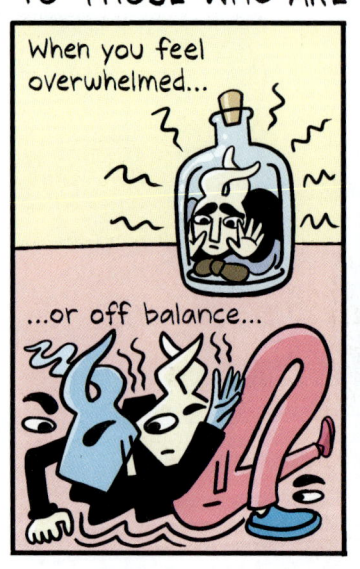

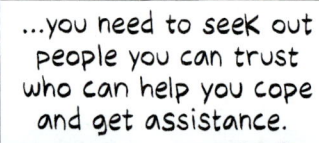

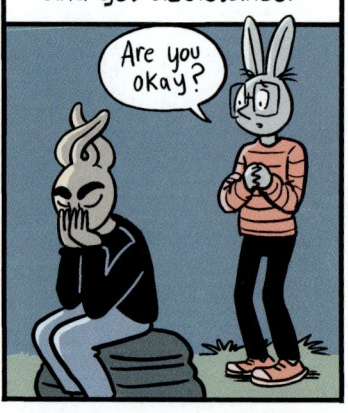

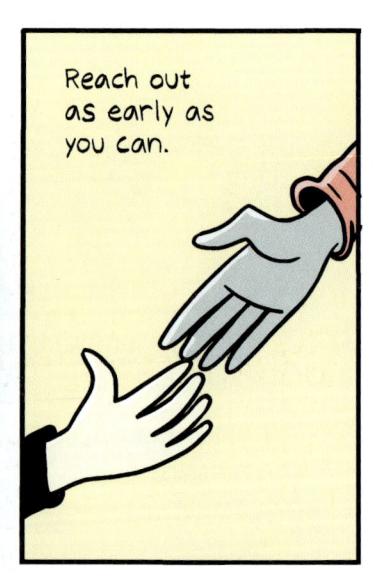

When you feel overwhelmed...

...or off balance...

...you need to seek out people you can trust who can help you cope and get assistance.

Are you okay?

Reach out as early as you can.

TO THOSE WHO CAN OFFER SUPPORT...

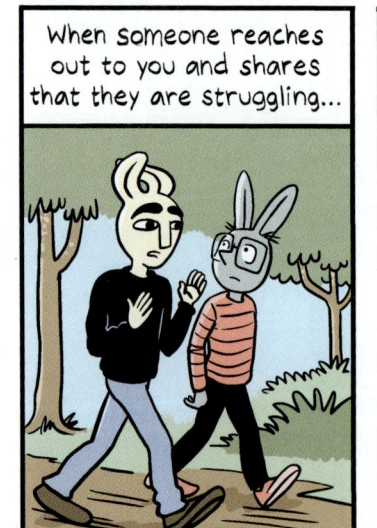

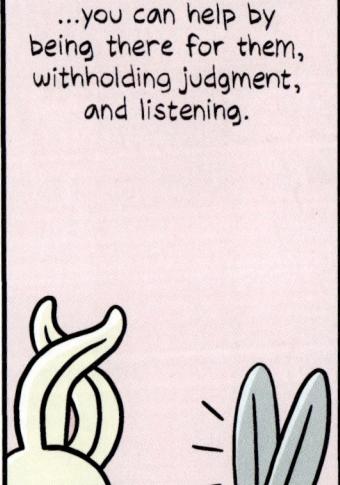

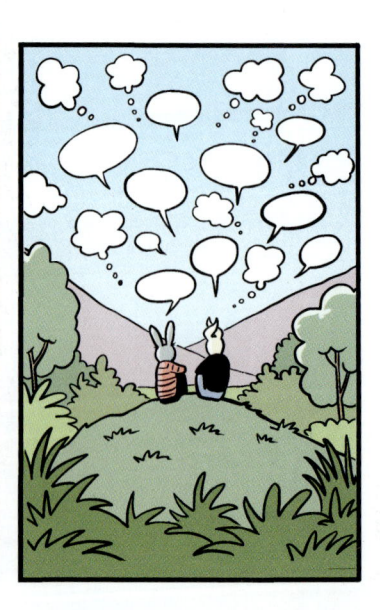

When someone reaches out to you and shares that they are struggling...

...you can help by being there for them, withholding judgment, and listening.